Botanical
Body Care

"An insightful, articulate, and eminently usable book! Karin Uphoff seamlessly integrates herbal, dietary, and lifestyle insights with her perspective on how the body works. This is a perfect blend of the practical and inspirational, and a welcome addition to the libraries of all concerned with holistic health care."

— David Hoffmann, MNIMH, author of *The New Holistic Herbal*

"I am especially impressed with the balance of this book: the diet and herbal suggestions, recipes, quotations, and especially the physiology, come together to create a holistic offering that fills a gap in the available herbal / health books."

— Donna d'Terra, herbalist, teacher, and founder of the Herbalist Mentoring Network of Mendocino County

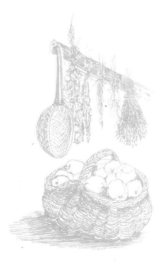

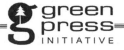

Botanical
Body Care

*Herbs and Natural Healing
for Your Whole Body*

Karin C. Uphoff M.S., M.H.

Illustrations by Emily Whittlesey

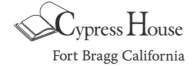

Cypress House

Fort Bragg California

Botanical Body Care
Herbs and Natural Healing for Your Whole Body
Copyright © 2007 by Karin C. Uphoff

Cypress House
155 Cypress Street
Fort Bragg, CA 95437
(800) 773-7782
www.cypresshouse.com
Cover and book design: Michael Brechner / Cypress House
Cover photo, botanical illustrations, and icons by Emily Whittlesey
Author's photo by Liz Haapanen

Disclaimer

The information contained in this book is based on the experience and research of the author, and is not meant to diagnose or cure. It is not intended as a substitute for consulting with your physician or other qualified health practitioner. Any attempt to diagnose and treat an illness should be done under the direction of a healthcare professional. The publisher and author are not responsible for any adverse effects or consequences resulting from the use of any of the suggestions, preparations, or procedures discussed in this book.

Library of Congress Cataloging-in-Publication Data

Library of Congress Cataloging-in-Publication Data
Uphoff, Karin.
  Botanical body care : herbs and natural healing for your whole body / Karin Uphoff. -- 1st ed.
      p. cm.
  Includes bibliographical references and index.
  ISBN-13: 978-1-879384-67-5 (pbk. : alk. paper)
  ISBN-10: 1-879384-67-1
  1. Herbs--Therapeutic use. 2. Self care, Health. I. Title.
  RM666.H33U64 2006
  615'.321--dc22

                                        2006001763

Printed in Canada
9 8 7 6 5 4 3 2 1

This book is dedicated to the memory of
Nilufar Zenouzi, who remains
as a flower in my heart

Contents

Recipes

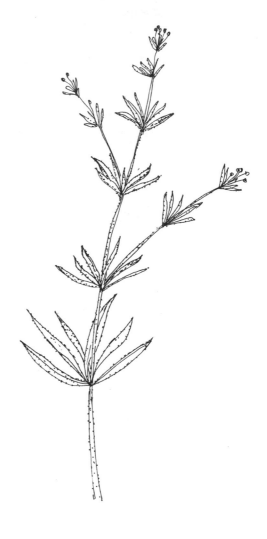

Acknowledgments

The ideas presented here are based on years of study and practice, and the legacy of great herbalists who have opened the path before me.

One of these great herbalists is the late Dr. John Christopher, of Salt Lake City, Utah, who dedicated much of his life to teaching patients and students about herbs because "every home should have an herbalist." Some of his students, such as Dr. Richard Schultz and Jill Davies, carried on his wisdom in combination with their own, and became my teachers. I also appreciate the insights and training I received from colon hydrotherapist and healer Cindy Sellers. Many thanks to all the students and clients who have served as my teachers — especially Emily Whittlesey, whose incredible enthusiasm and talents ensured the eventual publication of this book. My love and gratitude to Scott Roat for his constant encouragement and technical support throughout the many stages of writing. Finally, I give my deepest thanks to the magical world of plants, whose wisdom and gifts are infinite.

Introduction

The beauty, mystery and power of plants have embraced humankind from the beginning, as plants were here long before we began our walk on earth. Our partnership with plants is a fundamental relationship that continues to evolve.

We are far more chemically connected to plants than most of us imagine. Plants provide the sustenance for our existence and serve as ever-giving allies whose aid is always there — especially when we listen closely!

Herbal medicine does not use plants to treat symptoms the way prescription drugs are often used. Plants assist people on many levels at once, so that the underlying pattern of illness is addressed. Many different plants could treat the same symptom, yet only a few of them may pose a good match for the basis of those symptoms. Plant chemistry is intricate: how various chemicals in plants relate to each other, and how that synergy responds to the chemistry of our body, is the mystery of plant-people partnership!

Communication between the language of plants and our individual cellular intelligence can result in effects that aren't always predictable, thus there can be differences in response among different people using the same herb or combination of herbs. Matching plants to people takes more than knowledge of the plant: it also requires intuition and awareness of the subtle vibrations between the plant and the person. The healing energy of plants is further increased by the relationship we cultivate as we spend time with plants and use them for our health and well-being.

In the commercial world, health is often promoted as some ideal state of physical perfection, but upon examining the natural world, we find the true meaning of health to be more dynamic. Health is a *process* of balancing energy intake to energy output, and that varies from body to body and season to season. The ebb and flow of energy we take in and energy we release can result in the experience of *excess* (accumulation of energy), *depletion* (loss of energy), or *stagnation* (stuck energy). Traditional healing practices around the world address the root causes of excess, depletion and stagnation in energy flow, in order to free the body's own healing potential.

Taking energy into our bodies is nourishing, and we nourish ourselves with much more than just food and drink. We are nourished by the air we breathe, substances we apply to our skin, images and light through our eyes, sound through our ears, scents through our nose, and sensation through touch and temperature, etc. Our energy intake also consists of personal thoughts, feelings, beliefs, and values. Overall health is influenced by electromagnetic energy, relationships with those around us and the community and culture we live in, earth energies, energies of other planetary bodies, and solar and stellar energies.

Simply becoming aware of what you take in every day and receiving it consciously, both in food and non-food energies, can be very revealing. What are you allowing in that negatively affects you? What causes you to lose energy or triggers an emotional response? What do you put back into the environment every day, and how do you nourish the world around you? Do you feel a discrepancy between the two? Are you living in balance with your environment?

Even the simple difference between thinking or acting one way but feeling another can result in disharmony that manifests as an imbalance or disease (a state of dis-ease) in the body. As we fine-tune our awareness to internal and external cues simultaneously, we can make choices that create well-being and happiness for ourselves. Eventually, your choices will lead to feeling good about yourself, feeling at home in your body, and having the energy you need to meet the joys and challenges of your life.

True wellness requires an openness to change that allows for living vibrantly with a long-term outlook on preventive care. The journey of cleansing and balancing your body-mind-spirit, and addressing the intrinsic need for restoring your healing force and vitality, will renew the relationship you have with your body. This process of empowerment with the help of nature's allies is the crux of natural healing.

To address the nature of our body, we must work with it in a co-creative way. Nature has an intelligence that is not easily measurable, nor obvious except through experiencing it intimately. To come to the place where we can work *with* our body and all life forms around and in us requires that we listen to our intuition and heed our inner rhythms. Open to the intelligence of your body and how it 'speaks' to you. Allow yourself to respond to your body's natural impulses, while observing how your habitual mind counters those impulses. Spending time outdoors immersed in the natural world will help your mind settle into the miracle of your own existence. This book is meant to inspire you to inhabit your body with reverence, which will further your connection with the natural world and allow the magic of plants to open up to you.

How to Best Use this Book

The purpose of this book is to promote a basic understanding of how the human body is designed to function, and to provide natural healing tools for supporting our body's inherent vitality and ability to heal itself. Each chapter covers basic physiology of a particular body system, plus any applicable cleansing techniques and herbal remedies. At the end of most chapters is a more detailed section on treatment for common ailments. Exceptions to this are chapters nine and ten, each of which contain a list of specific herbs and their functions. Much of the material emphasizes cleansing and strengthening of the body using food as medicine. When we cleanse, we naturally peel away years' worth of cellular debris that is compromising our health and vitality — this is called detoxification, and is fundamental to healing and cellular regeneration. While moving out debris, we must simultaneously nourish the renewal of our tissues with high-quality foods and herbs that provide easily assimilated nutrients.

Because body type and constitutional strength vary individually, it's important that you always gauge your own cleansing process, the intensity of which can be easily reduced by decreasing suggested dosages and eating more lightly cooked food where raw foods and juices are indicated. Though many people have successfully used the formulas and practices described on the following pages, do not hesitate to tailor recipes or cleansing regimes to suit your individual needs and sensitivities. It can be of great benefit to seek the guidance of a health practitioner who has firsthand cleansing experience, and to enlist adjunct therapies to support you.

The quality of herbs and foods greatly influences their efficacy. Homemade tinctures of fresh organic herbs can be of better quality than manufactured preparations that use poor-quality herbs or those not processed properly. Plant chemistry is influenced by soil, growing conditions, time of harvest, parts harvested, and how they are stored or prepared for use. Often, your best medicine is locally and organically grown herbs and foods. Always scrutinize the quality of your herbs — especially if you buy them. Dried leaves and flowers should retain their color, looking bright, not burned. Fruits and berries should be sulfur and mold-free, and all herbs, including roots and stems, should be aromatic — just smelling them will cause a visceral response. Tinctures need also be aromatic, and the complex of flavors in the plant should dance on your tongue. Fresh herbs are nearly always preferable, but some, particularly roots and barks, rehmannia root and cascara sagrada bark, for example, are more effective when prepared (pre-cooked) or aged.

The first time a herb appears in the text, it is followed by its Latin name; otherwise, only common names are used.

This book is not an herbal, nor does it provide extensive information about medicine making. For this, the reader is referred to the many excellent books listed in "References and Recommended Reading." The appendices provide kitchen recipes, a list of the medicinal effects of cooking herbs and spices, a discussion of dosages, and basic herbal first aid. Also included is a source list for recommended materials.

Icons are used throughout the book to indicate the following:

 A cleanse that entails specific dietary guidelines.

 Drink mixes, usually in association with cleansing.

 A listing of specific herbs on the subject.

 Formulas that require powdered herbs or capsules.

 Herbal tea or infusion, also called a tisane.

 Decoctions in which herbs must be cooked.

 Tinctured herbs extracted in alcohol or glycerine.

 Recipes to prepare as food.

 Formulas that cleanse and flush specific organs.

Definitions and Preparation of Herbs

Tea / Infusion – Also called "tisane," is an herbal beverage using 1 heaping teaspoon of dried herb per cup of water (normally boiling hot), or 1 – 2 tablespoons fresh herb per cup. Allow it to sit, covered, for at least 10 minutes or longer. Tonic herbal infusions are made using double the amount of herb and are steeped all day or soaked overnight to drink the next day for maximum nutrient intake. Some herbs, such as flax and marshmallow, work well as cold infusions (soaking herbs in cool water for an extended period). Other herbs, such as usnea, are first brought to a boil and immediately removed from heat to steep, covered, for 15 – 20 minutes.

Decoction – A method of simmering herbs, covered, for 20 – 40 minutes in the same proportions as for an infusion. This method is required for most roots, hard berries, and barks, and may include overnight pre-soaking in cold water.

Tincture – An extract of herbs made by covering fresh or dried herbs with a menstruum such as vodka, brandy, apple cider vinegar, or vegetable glycerin. This mixture sits for a minimum of 2 weeks (1 – 3 months is optimal) and is shaken once a day or every few days. It is poured through a strainer lined with cheesecloth, and the remaining liquid squeezed out for use. Most alcohol tinctures can keep for up to ten years when stored in dark glass bottles in a cool place.

Fomentation – Essentially, an herbal infusion or decoction soaked up by a cotton or wool flannel and applied to a traumatized area as a warm or cool compress.

Poultice – A mixture of fresh or dried herbs and binders (vitamin-E oil, water, clay, slippery elm powder, cider vinegar, or saliva, etc.) that forms a paste which is then applied to an external injury, wound, boil, ulcer, tumor, cyst, or cancer. A poultice can remain on a wound up to 3 days.

Castor Oil Pack – Make by warming pure castor oil on low heat and saturating a wool or cotton flannel cloth with it. Place it over the area of you body you wish to treat, and cover with a waterproof material (usually a piece of plastic), then cover this with a towel, and place a heat source (hot water bottle or electric heating pad) on top to keep it warm for 20 – 40 minutes.

Botanical
Body Care

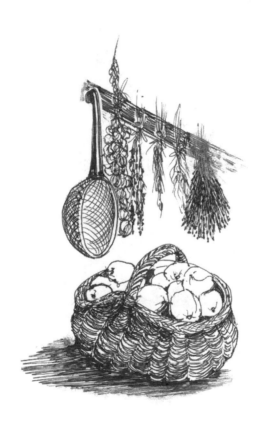

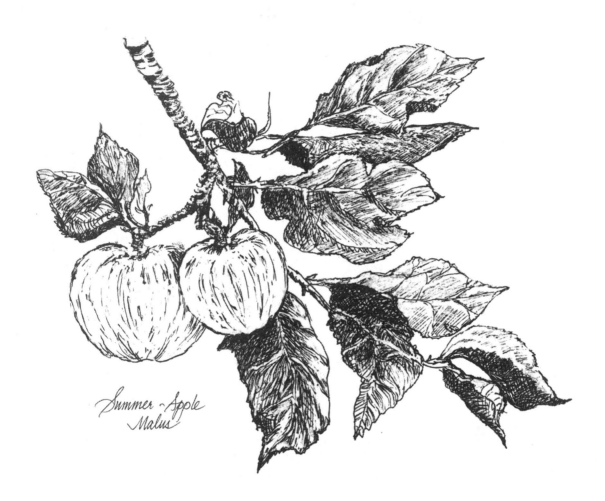

Summer Apple
Malus

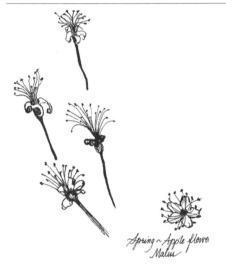

Chapter One

The Intestinal System:
Large and Small Intestines

Earth who gives to us this food,
Sun who makes it ripe and good.
Sun above and earth below,
Our loving thanks to you we show.

Waldorf meal blessing

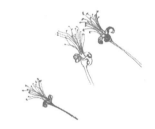

Imagine yourself crawling inside a damp, cool cave, twisting through tunnels of moist, convoluted earth of hard rock and soft mud. In this underground environment there are secret side rooms where stalactites grow from the ceiling, and places where the passageway narrows or widens. The intestines, the small intestine and the large intestine, or bowel, are akin to this deep subsurface terrain. Like the earth itself, our body, with the aid of water, absorbs and transports nutrients from the soils of our stomach to be rejoined with the substrata deep within our torso. Everything we swallow — food, medicine, pollutants, or feelings — filters down into the intestines, just as everything we throw onto the earth's surface eventually makes its way down to the deepest layers of the planet. Within earth's depths is an entire universe of water, minerals, and mysterious life forms that absorb, sort, filter, and decompose material, just as in our own bowel — full of creatures that never see the light, providing a service we can't see, yet which sustains us. Our own intestinal system is analogous to these open, active spaces beneath the earth's crust.

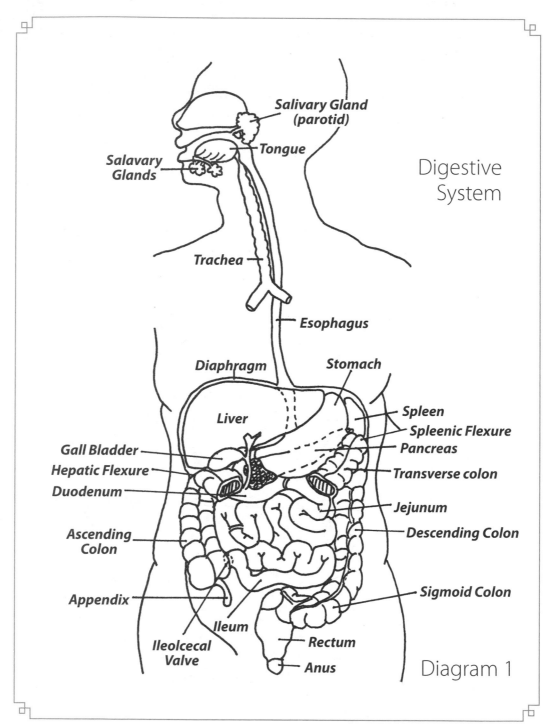

Salivary Gland
(parotid)

Tongue

Salavary
Glands

Digestive
System

Trachea

Esophagus

Diaphragm

Stomach

Liver

Spleen

Spleenic Flexure

Gall Bladder

Pancreas

Hepatic Flexure

Transverse colon

Duodenum

Jejunum

Ascending
Colon

Descending Colon

Appendix

Sigmoid Colon

Ileum

Rectum

Ileolcecal
Valve

Anus

Diagram 1

While in the womb, our large and small intestines are among the first tissues formed. Our tissues develop from the umbilicus, growing out in a spiral, like a young fern in springtime, and the center of that spiral is the intestine. Nature prioritizes the development of the intestines first, establishing assimilation and elimination as essential systems of survival, so that other systems may thrive.

A Gut Feeling

This primary spiral of intestine also has its very own nervous system, the enteric nervous system, which, though connected to our central nervous system, can operate independently. In fact there are more than 100 million nerve cells in the small intestine alone — roughly equal to the number of nerves in the spinal cord! The number of nerve cells in our entire intestinal tract exceeds the number found in the rest of our body. Every class of neurotransmitter in the brain is also found in the bowel.

Neurotransmitters are the words that cells use to communicate with one another. Serotonin is one such neurotransmitter, and most of the body's serotonin is made in the bowel; our brains make only 1 percent. Neuroscientists are continually amazed to find that the components of the enteric nervous system are more akin to the brain than any other organ — there is plenty of science to back up the term "a gut feeling"! Additionally, our intestines are the center of development for many immune cells, therefore an important player in the efficiency of our immune system.

Our life-force energy, or *chi*, is concentrated in the lower belly, located approximately two finger-widths below the bellybutton and referred to as the *hara* or *dan tien*. Traditional healing practices focus on exercises that strengthen the pulse of this point in which we hold our personal power. In the Ayurvedic tradition, this area is associated with the second *chakra* or sacral energy center — source of our sexual, creative, relationship, and life-force energies. In classical Greece, the navel or *omphalos* was considered the center from which we gather intuitive impressions and information, which are then sent to the heart, where decisions are made.

Healing traditions of many cultures have practiced cleansing and maintaining the intestinal tract. Interestingly, in modern Western society, this powerful center in the body has suffered ages of abuse and gluttony. Ignoring our lower center altogether tends to dissociate us from our animal nature in favor of the presumed higher energies of the mind; however, true enlightenment and mental clarity are more easily achieved when attending to the bowel.

The Small Intestine

Our small intestine consists of three parts: duodenum, jejunum, and ileum (see diagram 1, page 12), in which the breakdown of food and the assimilation of nutrients is its primary occupation. After partially digested food, or chyme, is released from our stomach through the pyloric sphincter, it enters the duodenum, which is nearly a foot in length. This triggers the release of digestive hormones from the walls of our duodenum and stimulates the liver and gallbladder to release bile. Bile enters the duodenum through the common bile duct and begins the breakdown of fats, while our pancreas simultaneously releases its enzyme-rich juices into the same duct.

The wall of our small intestine is a thin layer of circular muscle whose interior is covered with villi (tiny finger-like projections), which are in turn covered with microvilli, creating a massive surface area for nutrient absorption. Nutrients pass through capillary beds, which introduce the digested food into our bloodstream. The portal vein transports this food first to our liver for quality control and then onward into our circulatory system to provide every cell with nourishment. Digestion continues along our nine-foot-long jejunum, and finishes in the last part of our small intestine, the ileum, which is thirteen feet long and terminates at the ileocecal valve, the point after which our large intestine begins.

The Large Intestine

Our five-foot-long large intestine, also referred to as the bowel or colon, begins just after the ileocecal valve (below which hangs our appendix). It consists of an ascending colon, transverse colon, descending colon, and sigmoid colon. Each section of the large intestine corresponds to a particular area of our body, so that the nerves and nutrients passing through that section of the bowel directly affect a distant body part, in a way similar to foot reflexology, in which various points on the feet affect particular organs.

When intestinal contents are transferred from our small to our large intestine, they are essentially liquid. Some of this is water that we have swallowed with food, but a great deal more water is poured into our gut during the digestive process by the various glands and intestinal lining cells that secrete into the bowel. All pancreatic enzymes, acid, base, salts, mucus, and bile are delivered in watery solutions. In humans, approximately two gallons or nine liters of water enter the bowel every day!

Despite this massive water load, only about six to eight tablespoons (100 milliliters) normally leave the colon as stool. This means that our bowel reabsorbs nearly two gallons of water per day — a very efficient adaptation to life on land, as it allows us to recycle and conserve fluid. Even so, when feces are excreted, they normally contain 70 percent water to 30 percent undigested food and cellulose. It takes approximately ten hours for digestive refuse to travel the length of the colon, thus it can take fifteen total hours for one meal to pass through our entire digestive tract, the travel time depending upon the amount of fiber and water ingested. Fiber speeds up movement and absorbs the water that gives stools their bulk. When less fiber is consumed, fecal movement is slowed, allowing more time for water to be reabsorbed back into the body, resulting in hard stools and constipation.

Both the small and the large intestines are fertile gardens of flora and fauna whose bacteria alone can weigh more than five pounds! They cultivate more than twenty-seven strains of friendly flora — "friendly" because they are bacteria that metabolize waste products and remaining nutrients by converting them to useful substances such as vitamin B_{12} and vitamin K. Many bacteria work to neutralize toxic substances and other "unfriendly" bacteria, some of which can be so toxic they would quickly kill us if they entered our bloodstream.

The walls of our colon are thin, muscular, and elastic, and thus are capable of stretching in amazing ways. Internal pressure of waste material, specifically roughage, stimulates the enteric nerves, causing the muscles in the bowel wall to contract in peristalsis and move waste down towards the anus. Unfortunately, modern eating habits have tested the limits of our colon's stretching capacity! Refined "foods," saturated (especially animal) fats, hydrogenated oils, and sugars serve to create a sludge that sticks like glue, coating the bowel wall, impeding reabsorption of water. Infrequent bowel movements result in a buildup of this sludge and a backup of the fecal matter embedded in it.

The Dangers of Accumulated Waste

The longer waste sits in our large intestine, the more time it has to ferment, foul, and breed unfriendly bacteria, or become a nursery for parasites. This is similar to the way that kitchen garbage would fester if left unattended for weeks. As our bowel stretches to accommodate the waste, pockets called diverticula are formed along the wall, causing it to thin. Wastes can get stuck in these pockets for weeks, months, and *years*, leaching steady amounts of toxic substance into the bloodstream and poisoning nearby organs. When these pockets become irritated and badly inflamed (often due to bacterial infection), the condition is called diverticulitis. Since most of our total circulation passes through the brain daily (80 percent of our blood supply per day), it's understandable that cleansing our bowel often results in clearer thinking and heightened sensory awareness.

It is estimated that the average consumer in industrialized nations stores anywhere from five to ten pounds of fecal material in the bowel — material that takes up space and compresses other body parts. Additionally, impacted bowel pockets provide excellent housing for parasites (easily picked up in food) that rob nutrients needed by our body. Should the walls of these pockets thin, they are in danger of rupturing under pressure and spilling toxic waste into our tissues — often with fatal results.

Finally, an impacted bowel cannot perform functions such as vitamin production and cultivation of friendly bacteria. This results in nutrient starvation and depletion of the tissues. Basically, our blood is only as clean as our bowels. All that said, why suffer the consequences when cleansing the bowel is so easy? One of the best steps toward your own healthcare is to cleanse your bowel at least twice a year.

We begin cleansing and nourishing the intestines by stopping the consumption of mucus-forming foods that coat the wall, reducing absorption of nutrients and encapsulating toxins. Without having to deal with excess mucus, your body has a better chance to build and repair cell tissue. This necessitates what has been traditionally called the mucusless diet, but a broader version of this diet is referred to here as the Revitalizing Diet. For a more effective cleanse, follow the Revitalizing Diet for at least one week prior to, and at least two weeks after, bowel cleansing.

The Revitalizing Diet

This diet is designed to maximize our body's ability to absorb and reclaim nutrients, strengthen the immune system, and cleanse all elimination channels. By eliminating those foods that congest the lymph system and suppress immune response, we reduce the workload for our body. *All* animal products tend to congest lymph, bowel, bloodstream, and organs, and tend to trigger an inflammatory response in our body; therefore, *avoiding animal products* just before, during, and just after bowel cleansing is essential! Since only dairy, eggs, and meat contain cholesterol, cholesterol intake is eliminated simply by not eating animal products — this is particularly important for problems of the heart and vascular system!

The biggest problem with animal products today is general mistreatment of animals in the industry and the high level of growth hormones fed or injected into livestock tissues, along with large doses of antibiotics and vaccines. Growth hormones are used to force the animal's cells to grow beyond normal size and rate. These hormones are not selective for a specific animal, but affect *all* animal tissues — what do you think these hormones do inside of *your* body?

Growth hormones force the replication (thus expansion) of tissues, particularly those of the reproductive system (mammary, genital, prostate), leading to enlargement of glands and cancerous conditions in those tissues. Injected antibiotics and vaccines reduce your intestinal flora while encouraging antibiotic-resistant strains of bacteria to reproduce and survive in your gut and play havoc with your immune system. If you wish to eat meat, please buy carefully raised organic meat only! Fish is easier to assimilate and a healthier fare when wild-caught, but remember that our oceans are over-fished and contain high levels of pollutants (particularly heavy metals). Eat fish in moderation and avoid filter feeders such as shellfish and bottom dwellers such as sole.

If you're used to consuming meat and dairy, or associate such products with being strong and healthy, trying this diet will take a bit of mental adjustment. Remember that even the animals you eat depend on plants for all their nutrients. Green-plant foods provide strong life-force energy, since the photosynthetic process packages vitamins and minerals in a way that is easy for our bodies to assimilate. It's a helpful reminder that when you eat a bowl of salad, you're eating a bowl of sunshine!

Begin by eliminating the most mucus-producing foods such as dairy products and floured (processed) grains, especially wheat. Use organic rice milk, almond milk, soy milk, or water in cereals, soups, and sauces. When cooking with dairy substitutes, be sure not to bring them to a boil, otherwise they may separate — better to add them on low heat only. It's always healthier to cook food on low heat (below 300°F or 148°C), as it conserves more nutrients. For thickening soups, blend in cooked and pureed potato, soy milk, powdered arrowroot, or kudzu root mixed in water. You'll find that soy milk makes things as creamy as half-and-half, but you'll want unsweetened versions for cooking. For many people, soy milk can be difficult to digest due to its higher amount of lectin (protective) proteins as compared to other soy products. Where there is an allergy to soy, used soaked nut and seed products instead. Hemp seed and almond cheeses work well on pizzas, tacos, and enchiladas — don't be afraid to experiment!

Eating consciously and responsibly is what is important. What you eat is *your choice,* so when eating, choose consciously, feel good about the choices you make, always honor your body, and thank the earth. One way to thank the earth (and honor your body) is to buy organic, non-genetically modified food products whenever possible. By supporting organic growers, we make organic foods more available and help protect the environment. Though organic products may cost more in the store, they're far less expensive in terms of your own health, the health of future generations, and the well-being of our planet.

Remember that the prices of non-organic products do not reflect the true cost of production, cost of environmental impact (toxic cleanup and reduction of soil fertility), and cost in terms of healthcare. *Pesticides and herbicides kill cell proteins — including our own.* Think twice about eating poisonous substances! *Read labels carefully* in order to *avoid all refined, processed "foods," and artificial colorings, flavorings, and sweeteners.* Nearly all artificial ingredients are linked to cancer and mental illness. Highly refined flours, sugars, fried foods, sodas, and many "diet foods" cause oxidation (literally *rust*) in our body, which inhibits cell regeneration and vitality of the immune system. This is especially true of saccharine, NutraSweet, aspartame, high-fructose corn syrup, and other chemically made sugar substitutes, which are nerve poisons.

When you need a sweetener, use raw honey (not heat-treated), pure maple syrup, rice, agave or barley syrup, date sugar, grape sugar, stevia leaf, long dan fruit, or concentrated fruit juice. When using these sugars in recipes calling for sweeteners, cut the amount by one-fourth to one-half, since they are often sweeter than cane sugar. Remember that even though other sweeteners are easier to assimilate and healthier than processed cane sugar, *they are still sugar* (except for stevia) and it is better to eat less sweet and enjoy other flavors, like sour, bitter, and pungent — all delightful to the palate!

Salty foods are over-consumed and stressful to the heart and kidneys. Substitute by using seaweeds, Bragg Liquid Aminos, or small amounts of pure sea salt in your food. Substances such as coffee, chocolate, alcohol, and nicotine are acid-forming to the blood and degenerative to the liver, pancreas, and adrenal glands. They are powerful *drugs* and should only be ingested responsibly — they are *not* a part of the regenerative food program!

Finally, *avoid all hydrogenated fats* found in margarine, vegetable shortening, and many packaged cookies and crackers. Hydrogenated fats are more dangerous for your body than butter. Being subjected to high temperatures changes their molecular bonding; your body cannot process them, and stores them in the form of liver and gallstones and on the inside of vascular walls.

Cold-pressed extra-virgin olive oil and coconut oil are nutritionally superior and won't go rancid if stored in a very dark glass or clay container in a cool place. Sesame oil, sunflower oil, walnut oil, and flaxseed oil are also good, but must be refrigerated, since they go rancid more easily. Once any seed or nut is crushed, the oils are released and begin to oxidize, creating rancidity. Oils cooked over 350°F or 176°C are oxidizing (rob the body of oxygen). Instead, try stable fats such as coconut oil, macadamia nut oil, or ghee (clarified butter) for fast, high-temperature cooking. As a general rule, cooking temperature should not exceed 350°F or 176°C, and it is best to sauté in a small amount of water, then add oils after food is cooked.

A word about wheat, a staple grain of many cultures in its whole form: *whole-wheat grain* (usually sold as "wheatberries" or "cracked" or bulgur wheat) is an excellent source of protein and vitamin E, providing nutritional support for the heart and bowels. Add wheat germ (high in essential fatty acids and fiber) to cereals or smoothies (wheat germ must be kept refrigerated). Also good is tabouli (sprouted-wheat salad) and 100 percent sprouted-wheat, yeast-free breads (kept in the refrigerated section your health-food store). When wheat is processed into flour, its nutritional value diminishes, and the higher gluten content makes it irritating to the digestive tract, causing the body to produce mucus that clogs the lungs and bowel.

Many people suffer a mild allergy to wheat gluten due to years of over-consumption, so it's best to avoid wheat products altogether. Keep to all-corn tortillas, rice cakes, natural sourdough rye (or all-rye crackers), and, for baking, use buckwheat, barley, spelt, rice, or soy flours.

There are plenty of delicious things to eat! *All vegetables* raw and lightly cooked, *all legumes* (peas, beans, lentils), *all seeds and nuts* — this means 100 percent organic nut butters, such as cashew, almond, hazelnut, and sesame, all of which can be spread on crackers and used in salad dressings and sauces. Peanut butter is not recommended due to naturally high fungus levels or high pesticide levels used to kill fungus. Eating *all whole grains* (rice, millet, cracked wheat, amaranth, oats, quinoa, etc.), and *all fruits* fresh or dried, preferably in season, is satisfying!

Many vegetable proteins are provided by all the amazing beans, which can be sprouted for easier assimilation: aduki, pinto, white beans, garbanzo, anasazi, black, mung, lentils, edamame (fresh soy bean) or soaked nuts and seeds, brown rice, bulgur wheat, nut butters, and tempeh. While the whole soy bean is nutritionally superior, tofu can be used for sandwich spreads and dips, and firm tofu works well for stir-fry and taco or casserole fillings or can be marinated, braised, or broiled. Commercial tofu and hydrolyzed vegetable protein are highly processed products and therefore more difficult for our bodies to assimilate; consume them in moderate amounts. Tofu and tempeh taste the way you flavor them, so be liberal with herbs and spices. Tempeh is a very firm fermented soy curd; it's far more easily digested and is available flavored with herbs or smoked. Always buy non-gmo soy products (containing no genetically modified organisms).

We can enjoy a bountiful buffet of choices! The emphasis is on *variety* (don't just eat the same ten things), *freshness* (fresh and local organic foods) and *flavor* (use an assortment of herbs and spices, while putting plenty of love and joy into your food preparation). With tools such as a crockpot, food dehydrator, wok, rice cooker, steamer, blender, and juicer, creative food preparation is unlimited.

Back to Basics Eating

Here are some basics about eating, the chemistry of foods, and the mechanics of human digestion:

※ The first drink whenever you wake up should be a glass of spring water. Drink plenty of water all day — for cleansing, a gallon a day is necessary.

※ Always allow at least half an hour of "wake-up" time from sleep before you eat anything. In the morning, sip a hot beverage to prime your digestive system before having breakfast. Try the Good Mornin' Drink described in the appendix, or hot water with a little organic apple cider vinegar or fresh-squeezed lemon juice and a dash of apple juice. This will flush the kidneys, alkalize the blood, and balance stomach acids (remember to drink your water first!).

※ Eat when you're hungry; if you're not hungry, don't eat!

※ Start your day with fruit, nuts, and seeds, along with "super-foods" like blue-green algae, chlorella, spirulina, wheat, barley, or kamut grasses. Combine in a smoothie or take greens and fruits separately.

※ Wait half an hour after eating fresh fruit before you eat grains or legumes. It's best to stay with fruit, nuts, and seeds until late morning or noon if possible, especially in warm weather. In cool weather, or if you have sugar sensitivities, you may want soaked or slow-cooked grains, nuts, seeds, and vegetables for breakfast.

※ Make fruit a separate course / snack; do not combine fresh fruit and fruit juices with grains and legumes. Exceptions to this are cooked or dried fruits, orange zest (for flavor), and lemon or lime. Lemons and limes are alkalizing and help digest fats, so they can be sprinkled liberally on foods at every meal.

❋ Eat vegetables, whole grains, and legumes for lunch and dinner. In moderately warm to hot climates, a big salad with a variety of vegetables and proteins is fulfilling. Emphasizing raw foods at breakfast and lunch is very cleansing and energizing, and provides the necessary live enzymes for strong digestion. Promote healthy bowel flora by eating cultured foods (miso, *natural sauerkraut, rejuvelac,* umeboshi plum, *sunflower sauce,* and active yogurt cultures, or take acidophilus / probiotic supplements). A balanced dinner consists of 50 percent vegetables to 25 percent whole grains, to 25 percent proteins, with essential fatty acids as part of the mix. Do not eat dinner just before bed.

❋ *Chew food thoroughly and slowly;* much of digestion begins in your mouth!

❋ Take your time and enjoy your meal. Do not eat with the TV on, or if you're upset, angry, or rushed. Emotional states affect digestive capacity. If you don't have time to eat, then keep food liquid or easy to digest. Try a pick-me-up of soups, super-foods, vegetable juice blends, smoothies, raw veggies, fruits, or nuts. Once you have time to sit down and relax, you can eat a regular meal.

❋ Do not stuff yourself at meals. After meals you should feel satisfied, comfortable, and energized, *not* full, bloated, and tired (that is your digestive system yelling for help). It's generally better to eat small portions more often, especially where there are blood sugar problems. A comfortable meal size is what you can hold in the palms of your cupped hands.

❋ Try breaking the habit of wanting "sweet" after meals — eat something bitter instead (it will help you digest), or have a tea blend with a little licorice or stevia.

❋ Gratitude aids digestion! Thank the earth every day for the nourishment it provides, and thank your body for assimilating it. Trust your body's wisdom by listening and responding to its subtle impulses. Practice this by recognizing how food makes you feel both while and after you consume it.

Be a Consumer Warrior

Unfortunately, the health-food industry is subject to marketing fraud just like any other money-making business. Just because a box or jar uses words like "Health" and "Natural" doesn't mean the food inside it really is — read labels carefully. Be extremely cautious of terms such as "Nonfat" (usually packed with sugar and flavors), "Sugar-free" (often laced with chemical sweeteners) and "Fat-free" (which can be riddled with additives and sugar).

Be a consumer warrior: challenge the industry and demand the truth! A good rule of thumb (about eating and life in general) is to keep it simple. That means buying raw ingredients in bulk and making your own mixes and bases. The simplest things cure, satisfy, and strengthen. Start enjoying earth's bounty the way nature provides it, without needing complicated sauces, frostings, and processed additions. Use your body wisdom and intuition; if eating a particular food doesn't feel good, don't eat any more of it! If you're strongly compelled to try something, do. Then, after you eat it, be aware of how you feel, and keep a mental record of your reactions to foods. You'll find that your body desires subtle dietary changes on a seasonal basis, so go with that flow. Make food your medicine by liberally adding "herbal remedies" such as the following:

For the Respiratory System: rosemary, leeks, onions, ginger, honey, cayenne, thyme, sage, cinnamon, horseradish, nasturtium, mint, tarragon, black pepper, slippery elm bark.

For the Circulatory system: cayenne, garlic, chives, lemon, marjoram, mustard, cider vinegar, paprika, hawthorn berry, alfalfa, nettles, turmeric, sea vegetables.

For the Digestive system: fennel, cumin, coriander, cilantro, turmeric, nutmeg, caraway, ginger, anise seed, celery seed, arugula, dandelion, mint, olives, dill, black pepper, vanilla, cinnamon, allspice, cardamom, mugwort, fenugreek, artichoke.

For the Immune system: basil, thyme, sage, oregano, raw garlic, onions, cayenne, nettles, fenugreek, parsley, fennel, cloves, sea vegetables, bay leaf, elderberry flower, reishi and shiitake mushrooms, astragalus.

For the Urinary system: barley, red / black / blue fruits and vegetables, nettle, alfalfa, pumpkin seed, all squashes, all melons, lemon, ginger, fennel, dandelion, rosemary, cucumber.

These are only a few! When you've adjusted to this Revitalizing Diet (allow yourself a month if necessary), you're ready for a bowel cleanse (hooray!) and the renewal it offers.

Bowel Cleansing

There are many products on the market for bowel cleansing, but whether you design your own or use a commercial product, there are two essential parts that make an effective cleanse:

One part is a liquid clay and fiber mixture taken between meals (three to five times per day); the other part is an herbal mixture (usually in the form of capsules) to tone the muscle of your intestinal wall and help evacuate the clay after it has absorbed toxic material.

The clay drink should include most of the following powdered herbs: flaxseed (for anti-inflammatory oils and fiber), psyllium husk (an absorbent fiber), bentonite clay (to pull toxins off the bowel wall), slippery elm bark and / or marshmallow root (to soothe and repair the bowel wall), apple pectin (to neutralize heavy metals), plant charcoal (to neutralize bacteria), and fennel or anise seed (to reduce gas). When ingesting clay and psyllium, you *must* drink a gallon of water a day! Bentonite clay absorbs a tremendous amount of water as it takes up toxins, and can act as cement if you don't drink enough water while also taking bowel-toning herbs to stimulate peristalsis.

The bowel-toning herbs may include some combination of Cape (*Aloe ferox*) or Curacao (*Aloe barbadensis*) aloes, senna pod (Senna alexandrina) or leaf, cascara sagrada bark, ginger (*Zingiber officinale*), barberry bark (*Berberis vulgaris*), garlic (*Allium sativum*), chamomile, cayenne (*Capsicum* spp.), and Turkey rhubarb (*Rheum palmatum*). Herbs such as Cape aloe and senna can be rather cathartic. These herbs are taken in capsule form during your last meal of the day. Dosage depends upon your bowel's response to the herbs and how much clay you're ingesting. Always start with the smallest doses and gradually work your way up — this is true of taking any herb or food!

You can make your own mixture of bowel-toning herbs:

Mellow Mover Capsules

2 parts aged cascara sagrada bark

1 part each: barberry bark, Turkey rhubarb, Oregon grape root (*Mahonia aquifolium*), ginger, cayenne, lobelia (*Lobelia inflata* herb and seed), red raspberry leaf (*Rubus idaeus*), Roman chamomile (*Anthemis nobilis*), and fennel (*Foeniculum vulgare*)

Mix these together as powdered herbs and fill into standard "O"-size veggie capsules. Take 2 capsules an hour before bed, and during the day if necessary.

During any cleanse, it's important to drink three-fourths to one gallon of water, get plenty of rest, take echinacea to handle floating toxins in the system, drink teas that assist detoxification, and keep all channels of elimination open:

* **Your skin** – perspiration, exercise, baths, saunas, skin brushing

* **Your lungs** – deep breathing, aerobic exercise, fresh air, singing, and free expression

* **Your kidneys** – drink water with lemon and a pinch of cayenne, stay warm and rested

* **Your bowel** – should be moving freely with well-formed stools

Try the following general cleansing decoction.

Top-to-Toe Cleansing Decoction

2 parts each: dandelion root (*Taraxacum officinale*), burdock root (*Arcticum lappa*), and wild yam (*Dioscorea villosa*)

1 part each: yellow dock root (*Rumex crispus*), sarsaparilla root (*Smilax officinalis*), echinacea root (*Echinacea* spp.), and licorice (*Glycyrrhiza glabra*)

½ part each: cramp bark (*Viburnum opulus*), cinnamon bark (*Cinnamomum* spp.), clove bud (*Caryophyllata eugenia*), Turkey rhubarb, and juniper berry (*Juniperus communis*)

Prepare as a decoction and sip in half-cupfuls throughout the day, drinking the equivalent of 3 cups per day.

Aerobic exercise is a great aid to bowel health. This includes yoga, chi gong, walking, hiking, running, and dancing. The bowels and lungs work together to remove excess mucus from the body — clearing the lungs helps the bowels and cleansing the bowels helps to clear the lungs.

Herbs that activate our bowel include stimulants such as cascara sagrada, senna pod, ginger, garlic, cayenne, black pepper, elderberry (*Sambucus nigra*), chamomile, Triphala (an Ayurvedic three-fruit combination), and herbs of bitter flavor.

Herbs that tone our bowel include astringents such as barberry root bark, red raspberry leaf, Oregon grape root, Turkey rhubarb root, turmeric (*Curcuma longa*), wild yam, burdock root, yellow dock root, Triphala, and herbs of sour flavor.

Herbs that calm and nourish our bowel include demulcents and carminatives such as aloe vera, wild yam, licorice root, cinnamon, German chamomile (*Matricaria chamomilla*), cramp bark, turmeric, catmint (*Nepea cataria*) slippery elm bark (*Ulmus fulva*), and marshmallow root (*Althaea officinalis*), fennel, anise (*Pimpinella anisum*), coriander seed (*Coriandrum sativum*), soaked flaxseed (*Linum usitatissimum*), and herbs of neutral to sweet flavor.

Foods that moisten stools include carob powder (*Ceratonia siliqua*), soaked figs, prunes, prune juice, beet juice, fruit pectin, molasses, very ripe bananas, slippery elm bark powder, natural sauerkraut, rejuvelac, miso, fresh juices, vitamin C and magnesium, seaweeds, wheat and barley grass, acidophilus and water. And don't forget relaxation of all kinds, so let go of worries and stress and have *fun!*

The Basic Bowel Cleanse

A bowel cleanse can last anywhere from five to eighteen days, depending on how you pace yourself. If this is your first one, take your time, since this is a new experience for your body and there will be a lot of residue trapped in your colon. Once you're eating whole foods and cleansing more regularly, two to three bowel cleanses per year should keep your bowel from accumulating toxins.

While bowel cleansing it's essential that you follow a vegan (no animal products) menu and consume plenty of organic raw fruits and vegetables. It's not necessary, however, to consume only raw foods, as you must take into consideration the season and climate you are living in. Slow-cooked whole grains, legumes, soups, and steamed vegetables are fine; just be sure to have at least one raw-food meal a day. Fresh vegetable juices are highly recommended as part of any meal.

Do not eat pasta, breads (except sprouted manna bread), sugar, baked items, baked oils (as in granola), caffeine, alcohol, carbonated drinks, vitamin supplements (super-green foods and protein drinks with vitamins / minerals in liquid form are okay), or drugs (unless you *must* be on a particular medication). You may eat all-corn tortillas (but not the chips), vegan tamales, rice cakes, and all rye crackers in *moderate* amounts.

Two excellent products for bowel cleansing are American Botanical Pharmacy's Intestinal Formula #1 (ICF #1) and Intestinal Formula #2 (ICF #2). See appendix for how to obtain these. ICF #1 is used to increase peristaltic action, thus increase your number of bowel movements, while ICF #2 is a clay mixture that pulls old fecal matter out of bowel pockets and off the bowel wall. Begin by taking one ICF #1 capsule during your scrumptious organic vegan dinner. The next day, you should note an obvious increase in bowel activity; if you don't, then take two capsules during your evening meal the next night. Increase the number of capsules by *one* each night until there's a noticeable improvement in bowel activity. *Only then are you ready for Formula #2.*

One hour after breakfast (a fruit smoothie with super-foods and protein powder is recommended), place one rounded teaspoon of ICF #2 in a jar with eight to ten ounces of water and / or half apple juice and half water; shake well, drink up, and follow with another jar of water. For the first day, repeat the clay drink once between lunch and dinner and again one hour before bed, for a total of three teaspoons. Take the number of ICF #1 capsules you took with dinner the evening before, plus one more. The next day, introduce more clay by also taking it a half hour before lunch, and a half hour before dinner. Again, take the number of ICF #1 capsules you took the evening before, plus one more with your dinner. Find the dosage of capsules you need each evening based on the amount of clay you take (i.e., the more clay consumed, the more capsules needed) and the activity of your bowel. Stools should be soft, well formed, and regular (at least two bowel movements a day). If stools are too loose or you experience cramping, reduce the number of capsules by one each evening until the dosage feels right. If your bowels are extra-sensitive to the ICF #1 capsules, another commercial formula, or the Mellow Mover capsules described above will suit you better. A total of five teaspoons of clay mix may be consumed each day, but if you take less, that's fine too. Either way, you complete the bowel cleanse when you have finished your container of ICF #2 powder.

You need to drink a gallon of spring or purified water each day during this cleanse! Drink two to four cups of Top-to Toe Cleansing decoction or another detoxification tea daily to assist your liver in processing toxins. Due to the release of toxins in the body, it's important to take a small dose (twenty to forty drops, twice a day) of echinacea and / or lomatium (*Lomatium dissectum*). During the cleanse, bowel movements should come easily and often, as the clay mixture assists the movement of old fecal matter out of the system as quickly as possible. Once you've finished your container of clay, taper off on the capsules for the next two to three days as the rest of the clay moves through your system. This cleanse helps rid your intestines of chemical residues, heavy metals, radiation, some parasites, and candida overgrowth. Repeating the cleanse every three months for one year will help your entire body rejuvenate. It may also clear your mind, emotions, excess weight, food cravings, and backache or leg pain caused by stagnant toxins. By the end of your bowel cleanse, you'll find yourself feeling light, energized, and out of toilet paper!

Earth I am, fire I am,
Air and water and spirit I am!

—a nice chant while cleansing.

Help for Common Ailments

Appendix Pain

Some medical texts consider the appendix a useless evolutionary vestige. In leaf-eating primates, it was the site of a larger cecum, or sac, that broke down vast amounts of fiber. Now it is reduced to a thumb-sized sac situated just after the ileocecal valve, which stops contents of the large intestine from backing into the small intestine. The appendix harbors probiotic bacteria that both aid digestion and support the immune system. Recent studies have shown a link between a healthy appendix and immune strength. Unfortunately, it's a very easy place for fecal material to back up into and get stuck, especially if feces become impacted. Appendicitis is inflammation of the appendix due to impaction that has festered and become toxic. This problem is preventable by keeping the bowel moving and discouraging the build-up of waste material! Such impaction typically occurs at a very young age from eating refined foods, insufficient chewing of dry roughage (like chips or popcorn), and not drinking enough water, resulting in fecal backup and constipation. By the time one reaches adulthood, some of the oldest contents of the bowel can be petrified in this location!

Acute appendicitis can begin days or weeks before, as pain on the lower right side of the belly radiating down the inside of the right leg, inflammation and tenderness over the area, nausea upon eating, and even vomiting. Months before these signs, there may be slight discomfort, tightness, and pain at the appendix area in response to eating and drinking certain foods such as coffee, alcohol, fried foods, heavy proteins (nuts, chocolate, meats), or large quantities of roughage. These early warning signs say it is time to cleanse the bowel and to eliminate those foods that trigger discomfort. Supplemental vitamin E or wheat germ oil can be helpful at this time.

An appendicitis attack is indicated when pain becomes severe. *Stop* eating or drinking anything! **A ruptured appendix can be fatal,** as bacteria and toxins are set loose in your body. Use your better judgment based on your location and circumstances; call someone to take you to the nearest hospital, where a surgeon will likely remove it. Even as you wait, however, you can give yourself relief *prior* to appendix rupture by taking some emergency tincture (see appendix for herbal first aid) and by placing a warm castor oil pack or ginger compress over the area.

Make a castor oil pack by warming castor oil on low heat on the stovetop or placing the bottle in a container of hot water, then saturate a wool or cotton flannel with it. Lay the saturated material on the area of your body that needs soothing. Cover with plastic, then a towel, and place a heating pad or hot water bottle over the top to keep it warm. The castor oil will enter the skin and gently pull toxins down into the bowel to be eliminated.

If major symptoms have subsided and you wish to continue treatment at home, prepare water for a high enema, or better yet, have a friend prepare it for you while you rest and swallow one teaspoon of echinacea tincture.

Make 1 – 2 quarts of a strong tea of equal parts of catnip, chamomile, and two cloves of crushed garlic, plus a dropper of lobelia tincture.

Pour the cooled tea into an enema bag, adding warm water until it is full and comfortably warm to the touch. Hang the enema bag high and insert the tube while lying on your left side. As it fills your colon, roll onto your back, massaging the abdomen to loosen debris, and then lie on your right side, allowing the mixture to fill as much of the colon as possible. It might not get very far the first time, but once it travels as far as it can, get up and eliminate the contents — do not retain the enema for more than three minutes. Repeat once or twice until you feel relief as the pressure of the bowel contents is taken off the appendix. Then take forty drops of echinacea tincture every hour for the first day, then every three hours for the following three days.

Drink only water, herbal (decaffeinated) teas, and fresh-pressed vegetable juices for the next three days. Eat soft (cooked) foods, soups, and juices, and very few raw, fibrous foods (unless well pureed). Take oregano oil (*Origanum vulgare*) orally in small amounts (one to two drops in water or juice) if infection is present, as indicated by elevated temperature. Once all symptoms have subsided, you may embark on the bowel cleanse as described above. To most thoroughly address the problem, find a certified colon hydrotherapist who uses natural, gravity-fed (not pressurized) herbal colonic techniques (see source list).

Colitis

Colitis is characterized by inflammation of one or more sections of the large intestine and is one of the most common bowel complaints. It can be set off by intense stress, anxiety or fear, so de-stressing and treating the nervous system are central to the treatment of colitis. Absolutely avoid all substances that increase inflammation: coffee, black tea, alcohol, sugars, drugs, dairy products, cooked oils and spices like peppers and ginger. Vegetables and fruits should not be eaten raw in large quantities — better to cook them, removing seeds and skins. Make it easy on the bowel by consuming pureed soups, generally soft, steamed or baked foods, to baby your bowel until inflammation has subsided. Six small meals a day will be much easier to handle than three larger ones. Eating / juicing raw garlic and culinary herbs like turmeric, thyme, rosemary, oregano, marjoram, tarragon, dill, cilantro, basil and parsley will help prevent putrefaction. The following tea will soothe nerves, decrease inflammation and soothe bowel tissues:

Fragile Bowel Tea

Combine 2 parts each: red raspberry leaves, marshmallow root, shaved or powdered wild yam root (or you can add the tincture to the tea), and peppermint (*Mentha* spp.)

1 part each: flaxseed, fenugreek (*Trigonella foenum-graecum*), goldenseal leaf (*Hydrastis canadensis*), licorice root, calendula flower (*Calendula officinalis*), and alfalfa (*Medicago sativa*)

½ part each: lobelia, and valerian (*Valeriana officinalis*)

Steep, covered, for 20 minutes. Drink half a cup, between meals, 6 to 8 times a day.

With colitis, you may experience alternating bouts of diarrhea and constipation. Herbs like blackberry root (*Rubus villosa*), oak bark and leaf, and meadowsweet (*Filipendula ulmare*) as teas or tinctures are excellent for diarrhea, while yellow dock root, soaked flaxseed (just drink the water), and prune juice ease elimination. Bayberry bark helps renew colon-wall elasticity and peristalsis. Drinking aloe vera juice and comfrey leaf (*Symphytum officinale*) tea is excellent for reducing inflammation and promoting tissue repair. For a powdered herb mix to sprinkle on foods for fast relief, see the recipe under "Irritable Bowel Syndrome" in chapter two.

Constipation

Constipation can be the result of anything from poor diet and dehydration to emotional upset. It can also manifest due to liver stagnation, parasites, nerve atrophy or spasm, especially when the spinal nerves feeding the pelvic cavity are pinched. Since the bowel is literally about letting go, stress, travel, and resistance to change can slow or inhibit bowel movements. Constipation can be reduced by *drinking more water*, eating more fiber (flax meal, psyllium husk, soaked prunes, raw fruits and vegetables), movement, deep breathing, spinal adjustments, relaxation, and the herbal aids mentioned previously.

Diarrhea

Diarrhea is not necessarily the opposite of constipation. It can also result when constipation has become chronic and has produced distortion of the bowel wall, so that water is not reabsorbed and liquid contents simply pass through. Otherwise, occasional diarrhea lasting one to four days is the body's adaptive strategy toward ridding the bowel of infection by offending bacteria, viruses, or substances not recognized as food. In such cases, diarrhea should *not* be stopped with drugs (as you may experience relapse or chronic infection later). Instead, support the system with anti-microbial herbs and extra fluids — especially water and electrolytes. Crushed cloves of raw garlic in honey can be taken every three hours, and tincture of echinacea / goldenseal or Oregon grape, clove, wormwood (*Artemesia* spp.), oil or herb of oregano, thyme (*Thymus vulgaris*), grapefruit-seed extract (GSE), and neem leaf (*Azadirachta indica*) will all help fight infection.

Food poisoning from salmonella can be fatal and is much more prevalent than we are led to believe, so treat with tincture of neem *seed*, taking one teaspoon every four to six hours; this is particularly important if you suspect hepatitis A. Also effective are capsules of wormwood, or oregano oil taken internally as soft gel capsules or in juice. Grapefruit-seed extract is helpful, but is better as a preventative. The greatest problem is fluid loss; indeed, diarrhea is still one of the biggest causes of infant death, primarily due to fluid loss.

Make an *electrolyte drink* of warm water with 20 percent lemon juice along with raw honey, potassium salt (or raw apple cider vinegar), and a pinch of Celtic sea salt (you can also open a capsule of magnesium or calcium / magnesium powder); sipping constantly through a straw is best. For children younger than one year, dissolve four tablets of Dr. Schuessler's Biochemic Tissue Remedies (homeopathic cell salts) in water and add to a bottle of milk or a bottle of water with apple juice and a squirt of lemon. Homeopathic cell salts will also assist those older than one year; just dissolve the salts under your tongue. Raw, organic apple cider vinegar, sea vegetables, and potassium broth (recipe in the appendix) will also help restore electrolyte balance. Remember that your skin absorbs water, so mist the skin with spring water with a bit of vegetable glycerin — add a few drops of rose, peppermint, and lavender oils if you wish. Helpful Bach flower remedies are rescue remedy, oak, and olive.

Astringent herbs help pull the tissues in and slow the process of elimination. One of the best is blackberry root decoction; blackberry and raspberry leaves are also effective, as is white oak bark (*Quercus alba*). Meadowsweet herb, arrowroot powder (*Maranta arundinacea*), kudzu powder (*Pueraria montana*), and slippery elm all serve to calm stomach acids. Use the bowel-cleansing powder (ICF #2) discussed earlier by mixing one level teaspoon in a full glass of water and drinking this one to three times a day between meals. This will neutralize and absorb toxins while slowing down water loss by adding bulk to feces.

Diverticulitis

Diverticulitis occurs where weakness in the bowel wall leads to the development of a pouch called a diverticulum. These may be small and numerous, or grow large as tissue is stretched by the buildup of waste. Often, diverticula cause no apparent trouble, unless they become inflamed, which is diverticulitis. Once inflammation occurs, any fibrous material ingested causes intense pain. Even though a diet of processed foods without enough roughage is the cause of this condition, once there is inflammation, one must eat only soft foods. It's best to stay on vegetable juices, mashed banana with slippery elm bark, mashed yams, liquid super-foods, and pureed soups. Herbs such as wild yam, marshmallow root, German chamomile, aloe vera, yarrow, fresh comfrey leaf, and flaxseed water will help soothe and repair the bowel wall. When pain is accompanied by flatulence, add carminative herbs like fennel, ginger, or angostura (*Galipea officinalis*). Use Turkey rhubarb root or senna tea with spearmint if there is also constipation. Once inflammation has calmed, begin to slowly introduce whole food and gentle bowel cleansing.

Irritable Bowel Syndrome (IBS) is discussed in chapter two.

Worms and Parasites

It's no surprise that all living creatures have other living creatures living on and in them. Use a high-powered microscope to look at anything in the world and you'll see layers and layers of life. Nature doesn't operate from malice or judgment, even though we humans tend to take acts of nature personally. All living creatures are continuously adapting to survive and reproduce, and in the process, evolve together. Even parasites depend on the survival of their hosts — all life is interdependent in a very delicate and often misunderstood way. Worms, other parasites, and fungi grow in and on us, but our health depends on keeping their numbers down to a bare minimum. All indigenous cultures have used herbs and cleansing techniques to eliminate parasites, and many wild animals forage on *vermifuges* (anti-parasitic herbs) seasonally to keep parasite populations at bay.

We don't pick up parasites only when traveling away from home; there are plenty in the soil, in water, in refuse and waste, and on pets. So, it's imperative that we treat parasite invasions when they're obviously causing havoc with common symptoms such as distended bowel, constant hunger, hunger followed by nausea upon eating, restless sleep, bouts of diarrhea, and grinding teeth at night (all of which worsen around full moons). We need a regular seasonal cleansing regime to keep parasites to a minimum. Parasites will always inhabit the intestinal system and lungs first, since these areas are "open" to the outside; however, the life cycles of some parasites, if they go unchecked, continue in the organs (especially the liver), and can create serious illness, disease, and even death.

A bowel cleanse that includes clay, charcoal, and eliminative herbs, along with taking a worming tincture, is the first step; if symptoms persist, the next step is to undertake gravity-fed herbal colonic irrigation by a qualified colon hydrotherapist. Parasites, bacteria, and other "germs" need waste material to live off of — they literally starve in a clean, healthy body whose immune system is strong.

Nature has provided us at least as many remedies to parasites as there are parasites! Herbs with a very strong anti-parasitic effect are: raw garlic and onions, pomegranate bark (*Punica granatum*), manzanita berry (*Arctostaphylos tomentosa*), cascara sagrada bark, pau d'arco bark (*Tebehunia impetigosa*), papaya seeds, nearly all seeds and rinds of fruits and vegetables (especially pumpkins, watermelons, and peppers), the green hulls of black walnut (*Juglans nigra*), all wormwoods, like mugwort, rue (*Ruta graveolens*), chaparral (*Larrea tridentata*), quassia bark (*Quassia amara*), pennyroyal herb (*Mentha pulegium*), neem leaf and seed, and aromatic spices like clove, cinnamon, turmeric, coriander, cumin, mace, bay, thyme, oregano, tea tree, and bitter orange (*Citrus auranthem*) — to name just a few! If the flavor is highly bitter or pungent, the plant is likely to be trouble for parasites. Many of the liver herbs are strong medicine against them. When undergoing a major parasite cleanse, please first consult an herbalist / health practitioner, who'll help you set up a specific program and check your progress along the way while providing any necessary support.

To do your own thing, begin with the basic bowel cleanse outlined here, and, during your bowel cleanse, take three dropper-fulls (90 – 100 drops total) of Para-gone! tincture in warm water first thing in the morning and last thing in the evening before bed (it's quite bitter, so add a bit of juice if you need to). Take another course of Para-gone tincture morning and evening beginning six days before the next full moon, and continue until the fourth day afterward, for a total of ten days. All creatures are more active and grow during a waxing moon — this is a time to get rid of any eggs and new hatchlings!

 ## Para-gone! Tincture

2 parts each: wormwood, black-walnut hull (the fresh green hull is best for worms, the rotted black hulls are good for fungus), neem seed, and clove

1 part each: rue, pau d'arco, and chamomile, plus pure essential oils of cinnamon, clove, and oregano (2 drops of each pure oil per 1 ounce of tincture)

Many parasites are more active in hot weather or hot conditions of any kind, so temporarily avoid hot baths, electric blankets, and saunas, which will encourage their proliferation and activity. Laboratory testing for parasites can be disappointing, in that pathology labs are usually kept cold, so stool tests can come out negative because the organisms hibernate or die. To keep parasites from entering or proliferating in your system, make a habit of eating raw garlic, oregano, rosemary, and thyme. Avoid clogging, sticky, mucus-forming foods, foods normally high in parasites: meat (especially pork), uncooked fish, and unwashed vegetables, and wash your hands after touching animals.

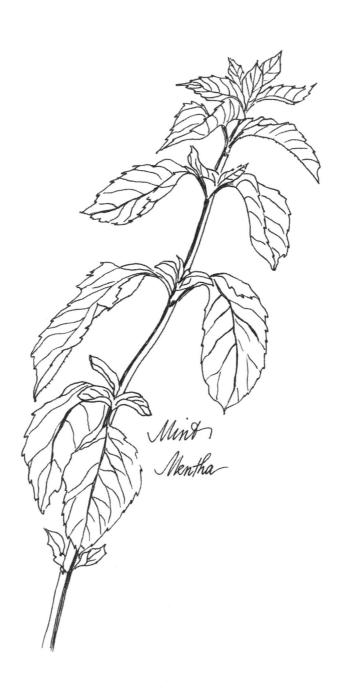

Mint
Mentha

Chapter Two

The Digestive System Part 1:
Stomach and Pancreas

The laughter is brightest where the food is best.

Irish proverb

When nutrients from fallen leaves and animal activities contact the earth, they are met with a plethora of microorganisms — a community of bacteria and fungi that vary with soil acidity, season, climate, and the other plants and animals they interact with. With the aid of decomposers such as insects, worms, and slugs, the deposited nutrients are broken down and absorbed into the earth to provide nourishment to plants, which then take up these nutrients and nourish us by offering the food and oxygen we depend on. Our digestive system works in a similar way, as the acids, enzymes, and bacteria break down the nutrients from our food, to provide us the energy we need to live.

Fennel
Foeniculum vulgare

Digestion begins when we first *think* of what we're going to eat and the mouthwatering aromas we *smell* as food is cooking. How we *feel* about our food affects the way we assimilate it as nourishment. For example, if you feel bad or guilty about eating something, your negative thoughts can actually make you feel bad as your body rejects the food on the cellular level. If, however, you revel in the delight of a favorite food, it's more likely to digest well. What we consume can bring us health and happiness if we've prepared and presented it with good feelings. Our eyes and mind feast before our mouths do, and any meal, however simple, can always look appealing!

Take a moment to acknowledge the beautiful bounty of your meal! How many *colors* does it include — the entire rainbow? Look at the *arrangement* of items on your plate, even if it's a humble snack. Stop to smell your food before you eat it; this sends your chemical receptors information as to how much gastric juice to make and what types of enzymes must be secreted, and essentially prepares the stomach, pancreas, liver, and gallbladder for digestive action. Contemplate for a moment the resources and labor that went into bringing you this food, give thanks, and *enjoy*! *Chew thoroughly* and *savor the flavor* (taste buds reside on the back of the tongue), honor food as your medicine, and *take your time* — up to 40 percent of digestion can be accomplished by relaxing and chewing food thoroughly! Mostly, this is the digestion of starches, with the help of the enzyme amylase produced by our salivary glands.

The Stomach

With the help of strong acids, and enzymes such as *protease* and *lactase*, our stomach initiates the process of the breakdown of proteins and other large molecules The most important enzyme synthesized by our stomach is pepsin, which catalyzes the breakdown of proteins into small components called peptides. Pepsin needs an acidic environment to work in, so the stomach produces hydrochloric acid. With a pH of 3, hydrochloric acid can dissolve metals like iron, burn a hole in any tissue, and kill most of the germs we eat with our food!

Our stomach protects itself from such caustic acid by secreting an alkaline mucus gel that clings to the surface of stomach-lining cells. This gel neutralizes acid and pepsin and prevents them from burning the surface cells just underneath. The lining of our esophagus, although quite tough, has no such protection. When gastric juice backs up into the esophagus by passing through the lower esophageal sphincter, the feeling experienced is heartburn or dyspepsia.

Additionally, the stomach produces a molecule called intrinsic factor, which is essential for life. Intrinsic factor binds vitamin B_{12}, which is obtained from food. The reaction of intrinsic factor and vitamin B_{12} produces an intrinsic factor/B_{12} complex that is not digested in the duodenum, but is recognized and absorbed by specialized cells in the lining of the last part of the small intestine or ileum. In the absence of intrinsic factor, the vitamin B_{12} we eat will not be absorbed, in which case B_{12} must be injected directly into the bloodstream or absorbed under the tongue. Vitamin B_{12} is necessary for the maintenance of many nerve cells of the brain and spinal cord, and vital to the formation of red blood cells.

The stomach is not an elastic balloon that squeezes back to size when empty. It is compliant in that it simply enlarges to the needed capacity — indeed a stomach gets stretched! Most adult stomachs can comfortably process about two cups of food, which may take up to forty-five minutes to move into the small intestine. Eating too much, too fast, overwhelms our stomach and slows digestion, often resulting in indigestion, un-digestion, or hiatal hernia.

Ideally, allow your stomach to "open" with a warm digestive tea sipped fifteen to thirty minutes before meals. To prepare the stomach and small intestine for digestion, try bitter or sour herbs such as Turkey rhubarb, artichoke (*Cynara scolymus*), rosehip (*Rosa* spp.), gentian (*Gentiana* spp.), citrus peel, or a tablespoon of apple cider vinegar in hot water. Helpful for awakening the liver and the pancreas are Swedish bitters (or an equivalent European bitters formula), or nibbling bitter greens, such as dandelion leaves, arugula, and endive, at the start of meals.

A healthy stomach is acidic when food is present. Many digestive complaints are the result of low acid production, resulting in insufficient breakdown of foods for the small intestine, which only accepts a liquid puree. Additionally, low levels of hydrochloric acid in the stomach often correlate with a poor immune system. Using antacids immediately after eating disables digestive enzymes, and therefore decreases the stomach's ability to break down foods. Eventually, constant use of antacids will stimulate more acid production because the sensor cells (G cells) in the stomach lining will notice the decline in pH and secrete gastrin, which stimulates acid-producing cells to secrete additional acid. Thus begins the treacherous roller-coaster ride of acid under-production when food needs digesting, and acid over-production between meals.

Certain foods can cause over-production of stomach acid. These "acid-forming" foods, which also acidify the bloodstream, should be avoided, especially for sensitive stomachs: chewing gum, sugar, simple starches, wheat gluten, hot cooked spices, such highly acid fruits as cranberries, kumquats, oranges, and rhubarb (note that lemons are alkalizing), caffeine, alcohol, drugs, and heavy proteins in animal products and roasted nuts. Avoid these also in the presence of ulcers, irritable bowel, and hiatal hernia.

Help for Common Ailments

Acid Imbalance of the Stomach

Balancing stomach acid over time is best achieved by following an alkaline diet such as that outlined by the Revitalizing Food Program in chapter one, and drinking apple cider vinegar and / or lemon juice in warm water each morning and before large meals. The malic acid in the cider vinegar will balance stomach acids and stimulate enzyme activity, as well as stimulate immunity and circulation, and gently open your bowels while flushing your kidneys. Cabbage juice is excellent medicine for unbalanced stomach acids and ulcers. Drink the fresh-pressed juice daily, or eat fermented cabbage (sauerkraut), which also cultivates healthy bowel flora. You'll find a recipe for sauerkraut in the appendix.

Acid reflux into the esophagus, also called gastroesophageal reflux or GERD is usually caused by malfunction or weakening of the esophageal sphincter muscle. Symptoms may be temporarily relieved by slowly sipping a mixture of a little kudzu root or arrowroot powder in water, or by sucking on umeboshi plum. A tea of slippery elm bark (or just stir the powdered bark into warm water), or water from soaked flaxseed can also supply some relief. Chewing on licorice root or deglycerated licorice tablets is soothing as well. Yellow dock root can be taken to reduce HCL levels. Strengthen the esophageal sphincter muscle with connective-tissue herbs (see chapter four), and repair tissue lining by using aloe vera juice, or the following demulcent tea:

Stomach-ease Tea

2 parts each: meadowsweet, chamomile, marshmallow root or local mallow leaf (*Malvus* spp.), and lemon balm (*Melissa officinalis*)

1 part each: slippery elm bark (finely ground), comfrey leaf, licorice root or fennel seed, red raspberry or blackberry leaf, fenugreek seed, and flaxseed

½ part goldenseal leaf

Steep, covered, for 20 minutes and drink warm (not hot) between meals.

The digestive enzymes and acids of the mouth and stomach are our first immune response and prevent bacterial invasion. To stimulate stomach acid, take Swedish bitters or raw apple cider vinegar in warm water, and enjoy more bitter and sour foods. As a temporary supplement, take pepsin with HCL just before meals. Foods such as sour apples, sauerkraut, miso, and umeboshi paste taken in small amounts daily will help maintain balanced stomach acids.

Indigestion

Indigestion is best prevented by slowing down and chewing food thoroughly. Eating smaller portions and not eating when upset or traumatized also greatly aids digestion. Choose foods agreeable to your body and combine them in a compatible way; refrain from mixing fresh fruits and grains. If your digestive system is very delicate or reactive, eat portions separately: first fruits / sugars, then proteins and vegetables, followed by grains or starches. In your food preparation, include seeds that reduce gastric upset, like coriander, fennel, caraway, cardamom, and anise. A drop of peppermint oil in water (or just the smell of peppermint oil) can provide relief. Indigestion is usually experienced after the fact, or as a result of physical pain, travel, or pregnancy, so keep the following digestive tonic on hand:

Digestive Tonic Tincture

Equal parts: chopped fresh peppermint leaves, grated ginger root, fennel seed, and orange or tangerine peel

Tincture in a solution of half brandy and half vegetable glycerin (or in pure glycerin if desired) for two to four weeks (the longer the better). Strain off the herbs, and carry this tonic in a half-ounce dropper bottle — handy for dinner parties or travel. Take 20 to 60 drops directly in the mouth, or in a small amount of water, as needed.

Irritable Bowel Syndrome (IBS)

Symptoms of irritable bowel syndrome usually occur in response to a trigger, which is often dietary or stress related — a strong message from your body that it's time to stop and get support in releasing anxiety and nurturing the self. One could also call it "the inner irritable infant" that is upset to the point of temper tantrum. Those with IBS have more sensitive digestive systems, and just after eating may experience evacuation of the bowel with cramps and diarrhea, the intensity of which is often related to the size and fat content of the meal. There may be an intolerance to foods such as wheat, corn, coffee, tea, dairy products, citrus fruits, or large amounts of fiber. Occasionally, infectious parasites (like candida or giardia) are involved, or there is a history of frequent antibiotic use. Herbs such as chamomile and peppermint are always appropriate for easing symptoms. For diarrhea try blackberry root (*Rubus villosus*) and leaf, bayberry (*Myrica cerifera*) or other astringent herbs.

Where there is irritation of the intestinal lining, such as in the IBS form of mucous colitis, nurture your bowel by eating soft foods, vegetable juices, pureed soups, and plain foods as separate courses. Keep portions small, and don't drink water, fruit juices, or tea during or immediately after meals; to increase digestive power, wait at least fifteen minutes after meals before drinking water or tea. Seed oils such as flaxseed, borage, or evening primrose, which are high in omega-3 essential fatty acid will act to reduce inflammation of the mucosa, and can be added to foods or taken as supplements. Make the following powdered-herb mixture.

IBS Powder

Equal parts of each herb, finely powdered: licorice root, cinnamon bark, marshmallow root, and slippery elm bark

Keep the mixture in a jar and use as needed by dissolving a teaspoon in warm water, sprinkling on vegetables or grains, or mixing into soft foods like applesauce, banana, squash, or yams.

To ease cramping take wild yam, cramp bark, lobelia, skunk cabbage root (*symplocarpus foetidus*), or black cohosh (*Cimicifuga racemosa*). Use one or more in combination with chamomile and catnip in a tea or tincture formula. Enteric-coated peppermint oil capsules do much to relieve spasms in the lower bowel. Herbs such as comfrey leaf, red raspberry, horsetail (*Equisetum arvense*), and the chlorophyll (green juice) of plants all serve to strengthen and repair intestinal lining. Bitter herbs such as wormwood, artichoke, or gentian promote appropriate digestive secretions and can normalize bowel function. B vitamins, which are particularly concentrated in fresh or freeze-dried algae, wheat, kamut, and barley grasses, are helpful, as is eating the right amount of fiber to pass formed stools or to ease constipation. Herbs like valerian, skullcap (*Scutellaria laterifolia*), and St. John's wort (*Hypericum perfolatum*), which treat the nervous system (see chapter eight), can be taken together with digestive herbs to address underlying stress. To identify triggers, record what you eat and any emotional situations. What in your life is difficult to take in, digest, or assimilate? Perhaps there's a need to slow down and process difficult information, experiences, or emotions.

Ulcers

Ulcer pain is described as a burning, gnawing, or aching sensation, often brought on by eating, stress, pharmaceutical drug side effects, low stomach acid, or lowered immune response resulting in an infestation of the bacteria *Helicobacter pylori*.

Prostaglandins and bicarbonate in the stomach naturally protect cells from acid damage; however, pharmaceutical drugs such as Ibuprofen (Motrin) and NSAIDs reduce prostaglandin production throughout the body, thus inhibiting prostaglandins in the stomach, and thereby subjecting the stomach lining to acid burn (ulcers). A bleeding ulcer can result in serious blood loss and should be addressed immediately by taking a level teaspoon of cayenne pepper powder in tepid water. Although using hot pepper sounds contrary to logic (the burning taste is temporary), it will efficiently stop the bleeding (being very high in vitamin K), is antimicrobial, and does not damage mucus membranes — in fact, it helps them to heal and move excess mucus. Taking cayenne pepper three times daily on an empty stomach (gradually working up from ¼ teaspoon cayenne in water or vegetable juice, to one teaspoon; or use cayenne capsules or eat hot salsa) will eliminate most ulcers. With ulcers, you first want to stop the bleeding and then tone and heal. Drinking one-half to one cup of fresh-pressed cabbage juice three times a day will also heal ulcers and may be more palatable. A safe natural herbal antacid is meadowsweet, along with herbs like comfrey, marshmallow, and calendula, which promote tissue healing. Discomfort caused by stomach ulcers can be relieved with the following formula:

Ultra Ulcer Tincture

Equal parts: bayberry bark, plantain leaf, slippery elm bark or marshmallow root, citrus peel, and mullein (*Verbascum thapsus)* leaf

Make as a tincture and take 20 – 60 drops with Stomach Soother tea.

Stomach Soother Tea:

2 parts each: chamomile, meadowsweet, and comfrey leaf
1 part each: hops (*Humulus lupulus*) and anise or fennel seed
½ part licorice root

Herbs that reduce infection by *H. pylori* are goldenseal, oregano leaf, bayberry bark, barberry bark, or Oregon grape root. Aloe, plantain, marshmallow, comfrey leaf, mullein leaf, slippery elm, and licorice will help repair damaged tissue and soothe the stomach lining. Other aids include spinal adjustments and "nerve foods" such as oats and oatstraw (*Avena sativa*), chamomile, mint, reishi mushroom (*Ganoderma* spp.), skullcap (*Scutellaria lateriflora*), St. John's wort (*Hypericum perforatum*), pasque flower (*Anemone pulsatilla*), passionflower (*Passiflora* spp.), valerian, and blue vervain (*Verbena officinalis*). Addressing emotions is also necessary, stop to take a look at what in your life is irritating or "eating at you" and make necessary changes to create a more soothing place for yourself.

The Pancreas (our "Sweet Spot")

Your pancreas is an endocrine (hormone-secreting) gland located just below and behind the stomach at the solar plexus. The major functions of the pancreas are to secrete digestive enzymes, which are activated in the duodenum; to secrete bicarbonate that neutralizes stomach acid, and to secrete insulin and glucagon — hormones that regulate blood glucose. The pancreas is "paired" with the spleen but works closely with the liver; in fact, pancreatic nerves are directly hooked to the liver and bypass the central nervous system. When our liver and pancreas are in harmony, there is digestive balance and strong "digestive fire." If there is disharmony, however, then blood sugar problems, inability to digest fats, weight loss or gain, nausea, and bloating occur. Our pancreas is responsible for making most of our body's enzymes by adding a co-factor to the incomplete enzymes it receives from the bloodstream.

Enzymes are proteins that catalyze and regulate nearly every biochemical reaction from hormone production to toenail growth. Most enzymes operate within a near-neutral (6.5 – 7.5) pH range. In fact, approximately 100 trillion cells in the human body depend on the reaction of enzymes and their products! Digestive enzymes secreted by the pancreas go into the lower stomach and small intestine to break down large food molecules. Other enzymes, called systemic enzymes, are released by the pancreas into the bloodstream.

Our body is capable of producing all the enzymes it needs, provided the necessary building blocks are made available through the consumption of enzyme-rich raw foods (enzymes in food die at temperatures above 118°F / 47.7°C). Raw foods actually contain most of the enzymes needed for their own breakdown — nature's built-in composting system! The more energy expended in digesting food, the less energy is available for producing enzymes that carry out cellular functions. For example, our white blood-cell count drops significantly for about one hour after eating as the body shifts into digestive-enzyme production. Enzymes from raw and fermented foods do most of their work in the stomach, whereas the twenty-two different digestive enzymes produced by our pancreas do most of their work in the small intestine.

Foods digest at different rates in acid and alkaline environments, so how you combine foods can have a radical effect on digestion. A general rule of thumb is to always eat fruits separately from starches and heavy proteins, although fruits, nuts, and seeds are compatible for most people. With the exception of bananas (which are very starchy unless extremely ripe), cooked dried fruits (like raisins in oatmeal), and lightly cooked or heated pineapple and papaya, the sugars and acids in juicy fruits slow the digestion of other foods. Melons are best eaten as a separate course because they digest very rapidly. Vegetables are compatible with both proteins and starches, but if your digestion is compromised, don't combine any heavy proteins, such as tofu or eggs, with starches.

There is no specific way to cleanse the pancreas, except to seriously limit sugar intake, balance the endocrine system as a whole, and generally strengthen the digestive system. A nice all-around toner for pancreas, liver, and kidney / adrenals is the three-flavored schizandra berry (*Schizandra chinensis*) taken as tea or tincture in combination with chamomile and a bit of lobelia. Many health problems, from skin ailments to poor immunity and joint inflammation, are linked to inadequate digestion! Spices to increase digestive energy include coriander, turmeric, fennel, cardamom, ginger, cinnamon, angelica root (*Angelica archangelica*), sweet cicely leaf (*Osmorhiza longistylis*), mugwort, nutmeg, and asafetida (*Ferula foetida*). The Ayurvedic formula, Triphala, will balance the upper, middle, and lower digestive sections with each other. It is a combination of three fruits in equal parts: amalaki (*Emblica officinalis*), haritaki (*Terminalia chebula*), and bibhitaki (*Terminalia beleria*), and is taken between meals and once in the evening before bed.

A number of factors destroy enzymes: cooking, pasteurization and irradiation of food, fluoridated water, pesticides, chemical exposure (especially chemotherapy), abdominal injury, drugs, and alcohol. Slowly increase the amount of raw foods and fresh juices you consume until your diet consists of 40 to 80 percent raw, soaked, or fermented foods (this varies by individual nutritional needs and season). Break the "snacking all day" habit so your system can rest and concentrate on enzyme production. Finally, *chew food well!* Even juices and liquid meals need to be mixed with saliva.

Sugar Metabolism

The average annual consumption of sugar in 1910 in the USA was about ten pounds per person. It is presently between 120 – 150 pounds per person! Our bodies have not had the evolutionary time to adjust to this recent historical (*hysterical*) trend. The best help for our pancreas is to eliminate sugar (especially sugarcane and high-fructose corn syrup, but all sweeteners as well) from daily food intake as much as possible. All sugars extracted from plant material are concentrated by the removal of water and fiber, thus they are far more quickly absorbed into the bloodstream than the sugars in whole fruits and vegetables. Rapid absorption of sugars causes a sudden burst in energy by raising blood sugar — much of which goes to the brain. This "sugar high" lasts until the pancreas rallies, pumping out insulin to lower excess blood sugar by converting it to glycogen for storage.

Once this happens, one experiences a "sugar low," resulting in lethargy, weakness, and depression. If exaggerated blood sugar fluctuations happen repeatedly, our body begins releasing more insulin for less sugar, resulting in low blood sugar. If sugar consumption is then stepped up to counter a low-energy feeling, a sugar-insulin tug-of-war begins! This will eventually lead to chronic high blood sugar as insulin-producing cells of the pancreas become exhausted. Chronic high blood sugar is what adult-onset diabetes is all about, so keep major sweets in the category of "festival food," to be consumed in small amounts at very special occasions. An alternative to sugar, stevia leaf is extremely sweet, but, unlike other sweeteners, does not upset insulin balance, and in fact may actually assist the pancreas. Read packaged-food labels carefully! Four grams of "sugars" is equivalent to one teaspoon of sugar. Six teaspoons of sugar cause an immediate decrease in immune response as white blood-cell production temporarily drops as much as 25 percent!

Help for Common Ailments

Hypoglycemia

Low blood sugar, or hypoglycemia, can be balanced by a diet of whole foods (no sugar, caffeine, drugs, alcohol, or "empty" processed starches). Eating four or five light meals a day instead of two or three large ones will prevent major blood-sugar drops that can leave you shaky, anxious, and disoriented. Take digestive enzymes in the form of papaya, pineapple, sprouts, and / or supplemental plant enzymes. Remember that raw fruits and vegetables are key. Foods that assist by strengthening the pancreas are sea vegetables, artichoke, dandelion, fenugreek, bee pollen, nettle (*Urtica dioica*), reishi and shiitake mushrooms (*Lentinula edodes*), fringe tree bark (*Chionanthus virginicus*), nutritional yeast (and any other foods high in B vitamins), cinnamon, allspice, cloves, bay leaf, basil (*Ocimum basilicum*), foods high in vitamin C, and algae. Foods high in chromium, such as mushrooms, hibiscus flower (*Hibiscus sabdariffa*), and Brazil nuts, can be eaten daily. A chromium supplement of up to 200iu / day can be of great value where hypoglycemia is severe. Aerobic exercise and specific yoga postures also balance the pancreas.

Hyperglycemia

High blood sugar, or hyperglycemia, requires the same dietary precautions, and responds to herbs such as devil's club (*Oplopanax horridus*), cedar berry (*Cedrus* spp.), juniper berry, black current (*Ribis nigrum*), bilberry, blackberry, and blueberry or huckleberry leaves (*Vaccinium* spp.). Excess sugar in the bloodstream is highly oxidizing to our tissues, causing cell damage and deterioration of nerves. Herbs and vitamins that diminish the amount of revolving blood sugar are Vitamin C (1 – 3 gm / day as a liquid is best), vitamin E, bitter melon (*Momordica charantia*), nopal cactus / prickly-pear cactus leaves (*Opuntia streptocantha*), *Gymnena sylvestre* (an Ayurvedic herb that also helps with craving something sweet), stevia, holy basil / tulsi (*Ocimum sanctum*), rosemary (*Rosmarinus officinalis*), onion (*Allium cepa*), eucalyptus (*Eucalyptus globulus*) and all antioxidant supplement combinations that include selenium, alpha lipoic acid (found in vegetables like potatoes), or pycnogenol (derived from pine bark). Remember that *breathing fresh air* is still the best antioxidant — and it's free! Other helpful herbs include mugwort, burdock, blue cohosh (*Caulophylum thalcatroides*), pine needle (*Pinus* spp.), chicory (*Cichorium intybus*), celery (*Apium graveolens*), centuary plant (*Agave americana*), cranesbill (*Geranium maculatum*), fennel, fenugreek, lemon, licorice root, nettle, oatstraw, olive leaf (*Olea europaea*), raspberry leaf, sage (*Salvia* spp.), figwort (*Scrofularia nodosa*), caraway (*Carum carvi*), and essential oils of thyme, vetiver, ylang ylang, and bergamot, used externally.

Syndrome X

Syndrome X (hyperinsulinemia or insulin resistance) is a group of metabolic disturbances that lead to poor sugar management by the body. This results from a genetic susceptibility and / or lifestyle factors such as diet, exercise, and stress. At least 25 percent of adults in the USA have this syndrome, as do many children. It is essentially a pre-diabetic condition. High insulin levels in the blood promote fat deposition, increased inflammation, increase estrogen levels, speed tumor growth, and cause oxidative stress on the body. Syndrome X is almost exclusively linked to a diet of highly refined carbohydrates (processed foods, sodas, and alcohol), heated or hardened polyunsaturated oils (fried, baked foods), low fiber intake, and lack of exercise. The above factors may set off a genetic propensity for this condition.

Insulin resistance eventually leads to adult-onset diabetes. Besides major lifestyle changes, the following natural allies can help: milk thistle (*Silybum mariana*), garlic, green tea (steeped no more than four minutes in very warm but not boiling-hot water), nopal cactus, bitter melon, hibiscus flower, bay leaf (*Laurus nobilis*), holy basil / tulsi, cinnamon, cloves, garcinia fruit (*Garcinia mangostana*), reishi mushroom, and all raw seeds. Supplementation with alpha-lipoic acid, chromium, selenium, magnesium, vanadium, and zinc is helpful.

Diabetes

Diabetes is a serious condition and is increasing at an alarming rate in the USA. *Diabetes A* is a hereditary condition in which pancreatic cells are unable to produce enough, or any, insulin. Syndrome X leads to *Diabetes B* (adult-onset diabetes), which is entirely preventable through dietary and lifestyle changes, although some medical procedures, such as chemotherapy or radiation, can cause it.

The following formula pampers the pancreas by helping to restore insulin-producing cells. Use it consistently along with other healing methods.

Pancreatic Powerhouse Formula

8 parts cedar berry

½ part each: mullein leaf, uva ursi, licorice, cayenne pepper, and barberry bark

Take as capsules or tincture at standard dose (see appendix) 3 times a day, 6 days a week, for 3 months or more.

Other herbs that assist in recovering pancreatic function are devil's club, jambul seed (*Syzgium jambolanum*), blueberry leaf, and dandelion. Try the following formula to strengthen pancreatic function.

Pamper the Pancreas Formula

Equal parts: hibiscus flower, nettle, finely ground dandelion root, finely ground elecampane root (*Inula helenium*), red raspberry leaf, burdock root, and blueberry or huckleberry leaf

Take six days a week at standard dose, as a tea, tincture, or capsules, while also cleansing the bowel, then liver, and making any necessary lifestyle changes.

"Fire Breath" and other yogic breathing techniques, abdominal exercises, sounding, and singing, all strengthen the diaphragm, which supports all digestive organs. Since the pancreas is one of our Solar Plexus organs, we strengthen ourselves greatly when we treat it with care, which basically means "all things in moderation"! It is also where our ego is connected to others in relationships. A healthy balance of giving and receiving in relationship to others and the universe affirms one's sense of self and thus this energy center.

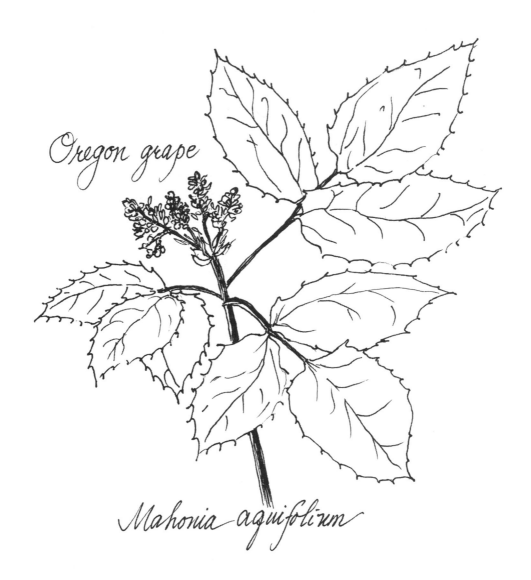

Oregon grape

Mahonia aquifolium

Chapter Three

The Digestive System, Part 2:
Liver and Gallbladder

May the beauty you are be what you do.

Possibly no other group of living organisms is so crucial to our life on earth as the plant kingdom. Plants take up minerals from the soil, air, and water, break them down, use them to nourish themselves, and transform them into the sugars, proteins, antioxidants, solvent minerals, and vitamins that provide animals the nutrients essential for life. Since plants do this with the aid of solar and lunar light energies, they are also harbingers of these energies for our tissues. Plants of all kinds also serve to detoxify our atmosphere, our soils, and our oceans. In this sense, forests, oceans, the bush, meadows, and green spaces are to the earth as the liver and gallbladder are to our bodies. Our liver and gallbladder work together to break down, transform, and store crucial nutrients, while disarming toxins.

Dandelion
Taraxacum officinale

The Liver

Located on the right side of the torso, just underneath our ribs (see diagram 1, page 12), the liver, weighing about three pounds, is our largest internal organ and is directly or indirectly involved in all physiological processes. Our liver is concave in shape so as to accommodate the stomach, duodenum, hepatic flexure of the colon, right kidney, and adrenal gland. All blood, containing the end products of digestion, passes through the liver before entering general circulation to the rest of the body. Thus, our liver distributes blood, regulating its flow to other organs, and sending nourishment to connective tissue.

The word "liver" hints at its function: "to live," and indeed we can't live long without this amazing organ! It acts as a defensive barrier between the things we take into our body and what gets into our bloodstream, cleansing our blood and protecting us every day from fatal toxins. In traditional healing, the liver is considered the home of one's will, and is subject to the emotions of a frustrated will, particularly anger, jealousy, envy, rage, and depression. A healthy liver works with our spirit to direct our life force in a positive way, and serves to harmonize our overall energy.

Our liver is a life-force source of energy because it metabolizes proteins, fats, and carbohydrates, and stores excess glucose as glycogen for the maintenance of blood-sugar levels. It also processes and stores B vitamins (especially B12), fat-soluble vitamins such as A, D, E, and K, plus minerals such as selenium, iron, and manganese. Our liver converts amino acids in order to make important antioxidants like glutathione, SAM-e (s-adenosylmethionine), and SOD (superoxide dismutase). It creates serum proteins like gammaglobulin (IgG, IgA) that are important for the immune system. It produces the cholesterol our body needs to capture Vitamin D, make steroid hormones (sex hormones), and make lipoproteins like HDL (High Density Lipoproteins), which transport fat in our blood. It also breaks down and inactivates excess hormones such as estradiol, estrogen, testosterone, and androgens, while storing red and white blood cells.

Our liver recycles the iron in the hemoglobin from worn-out red blood cells, and stores it for later use or turns it into bile, which contains bilirubin, a yellow-orange pigment caused by recycled iron. Bile is a digestive juice stored and released by the gallbladder for emulsifying fats and stimulating peristalsis, while also serving as a natural laxative and digestive antiseptic. As our major blood-purifying organ, the liver produces enzymes to convert poisons into harmless chemicals, and then eliminates them via bile that flows into the gallbladder and eventually out the bowel. Since the liver is connected with many other body functions, any imbalance in our body will affect the liver. Likewise, any liver dysfunction may manifest as a symptom elsewhere in the body.

The Gallbladder

Our gallbladder is a small pear-shaped sac wedged into the underside of the right lobe of the liver. It concentrates bile by first removing water and then releasing the remaining fluid through the cystic duct. Whereas our liver is the receiver, transformer, and protector, the gallbladder complements, taking the role of mover and manifester that pushes the energy and bile out into our body to stimulate functions. The cystic duct joins the hepatic duct from the liver to create the common bile duct, which empties into the duodenum. When the bile duct contains too much cholesterol, the cholesterol cannot be kept in solution and is not eliminated. Instead it forms hard stones, which block the ducts. When gallstones are large and numerous, they cause symptoms such as sharp pains just under the ribs on the right side of the torso, nausea, inability to tolerate fatty or fried foods, and diarrhea alternating with constipation and headaches.

The gallbladder is the primary outlet for the release of toxins from the liver. A *partial* list of toxins our liver tackles every day includes butadiene (in rug pads, rubber, petrol, car exhaust, groundwater), benzenes (in plastics and cigarette smoke), chlorine, DEHP (diethylhexyl-phthalate, in plastics and food wraps), dioxins (in pesticides and groundwater worldwide), ethylene oxide (gassed into herbs, coffees, and teas imported into the USA), glycol esters (in antifreeze, paint, sealants, ink, circuit boards), nitrosamines (in baby pacifiers, soaps, cosmetics, food containers), styrene (in water bottles, food containers, paper), trichloroethylene (in dry-cleaning fluids, paint, glue, insecticides), PCBs (in paints, plastics, furniture protectors), PVCs (in household and water irrigation pipes, vinyl, spray paints) — to name just a few! — and your liver is saying *Phew!*

Add to this what we might be putting into our bodies knowingly, like alcohol, drugs, pesticides, food additives, preservatives, rancid oils, plus parasites, bacteria, and viruses! Our liver and gallbladder are miracle workers! Common sense tells us that the more toxins we consume or expose ourselves to, the harder our liver must work. Our body has evolved a complex set of reactions to process common toxins such as ammonia, which is an alkaline gas, and the most toxic byproduct of a high-protein (particularly animal protein) diet. It is also a byproduct of pharmaceutical sedatives, tranquilizers, anesthetics, analgesics, and diuretics. Ammonia must be absorbed into the intestines and then whisked off to the liver to be converted into urea, which is then excreted by the kidneys.

Our body, however, *cannot* adequately process most modern chemicals, so the liver simply encapsulates them to protect us. These encapsulations result in liver stones that block blood vessels in the liver, rendering it far less able to perform its many functions. Those experiencing cancer and other serious diseases may have had a sick liver three to five years beforehand. When our liver is overwhelmed, toxic, and congested, we become weak and imbalanced, and the body starts to shut down. Periodic cleansing of our liver and gallbladder is necessary for everybody: if you observe animals in nature, you'll see how they naturally cleanse their bowel and liver twice a year, when seasonal vegetation provides the means, by eating plants that naturally elicit their bodies' cleansing response. Where winters are more pronounced, the need for cleansing internal organs becomes even more necessary, as rich winter foods and cold climate lead to hibernation and blood stagnation.

Basic Care of Your Liver and Gallbladder

Our liver and gallbladder can be supported by the use of hepatic herbs, those that stimulate liver function, such as barberry root, Oregon grape root, yellow dock root, dandelion, agrimony (*Agrimonia eupatoria*), fringe tree bark, bulpleurum (*Bulpleurum falcatum*), and wild yam. The traditional use of bitters or "spring tonics" was to tone and cleanse the liver and gallbladder after a winter of heavy foods and reduced activity. Bitters such as artichoke leaf and thistle, gentian (*Gentiana lutea*), sweet annie (*Absinthe annua*), mugwort, and chicory all work together to this end. When there are problems with liver and gallbladder function, it is crucial to avoid fatty and roasted foods and reduce all fats to a minimum. Taking small doses of bitter tonics daily before meals will maintain healthy liver-gallbladder function.

Care of our liver means being mindful of what we consume, including observing the general state of our living environment in terms of air quality, water quality, and overall toxic exposure (remember that emotions can be toxic too). Fortunately, this vast organ has amazing regenerative capacity and is quite easy to clean!

Eliminating pesticides, food additives, and hydrogenated and baked oils from the diet is the first step. The next is to take inventory of all chemicals in one's living environment. Replace traditional cleansers, soaps, shampoos, perfumes, garden supplies, disinfectants, and other household chemicals with less volatile alternatives. By using only biodegradable products, we feed the earth only what we feel is safe to feed ourselves. By doing so, we will stop poisoning both our own body and the planet's.

When toxic substances must be used (as in the case of most paints, for example), be sure to use protection from exposure by covering skin and working in a well-ventilated environment. Always dispose of toxic products properly as hazardous waste.

To mitigate the effects of chemical use, begin by cleansing your bowel. Always cleanse the bowel before cleansing the liver, unless it is urgent, such as with symptoms of gallstones, toxic exposure, and cancer, in which case the bowel and liver can be cleansed simultaneously. Once the bowel is cleansed, some liver flushing can follow as soon afterward as possible. Flushing your liver helps clear your gallbladder too!

Basic Liver Flush

This gentle liver cleanse is good for preventive care and can be carried out in the winter (cold weather), and by children over ten years of age, or those convalescing from illness. Follow this for ten days seasonally, or try it ten days on and four days off for extended periods to diminish toxic load, excess cholesterol, and liver or gallstones.

Classic Liver-flush Drink

1 cup apple juice *or* grapefruit juice, plus one cup water

Juice of 1 lemon or lime

1 – 4 cloves of fresh garlic (increase slightly each day)

½ – 1 inch fresh pressed ginger root *or* ¼ – 1 teaspoon dried ginger powder

1 – 3 tablespoons cold-pressed extra-virgin olive oil (increase daily)

A pinch of cayenne pepper

Stir together or put in blender and drink it each morning before eating. Fifteen minutes later, follow this with two cups of the liver-support decoction below.

 # Liver-support Decoction

2 parts each: dandelion root, burdock root, bulpleurum, milk thistle seed, and roasted chicory root

1 part each: licorice root and orange peel

¼ part crushed cardamom seed (*Elettaria cardamomum*)

Prepare as a decoction by bringing to a boil, then cover and simmer, low, 20 – 30 minutes. Sip slowly, imagining your liver as strong and clear.

Do not eat for one to two hours from flush time. When ready to eat, start with raw or cooked fruit, then half an hour or more later, vegetables (raw or streamed), whole grains, easily digested legumes (sprouted or slow-cooked lentils, peas, mung beans, or aduki beans), and fresh vegetable juices plus **lots of water**. During the basic flush, as in all cleansing, follow the regenerative diet as outlined in chapter one. Pimples, rashes, itchiness, or boils exuding from your skin are signs of waste products attempting to exit your body. This means you must further open elimination channels (see more details below).

If you'd like to jump right into more vigorous liver cleansing, try the following:

One-week Liver Cleanse

Most people benefit from doing this five to seven-day liver cleanse twice annually, spring and fall, which are natural liver-active times due to shifting energies and changing seasons. A bowel cleanse must be undertaken within one month prior to the liver cleanse, ensuring that toxins move out of the body swiftly. If, however, you are experiencing chronic skin problems, hormonal imbalance, constipation, pain or dullness on the right side of the abdomen, or other symptoms of toxicity, then your may choose to cleanse the liver immediately. If you do, be sure to cleanse the bowel simultaneously by using 1 teaspoon of clay mixture (such as ICF #2) one to two times a day to capture toxins, along with herbs to assist with their rapid removal. Get on the Revitalizing Diet one week prior to liver cleansing (if you haven't already). Some people like to alter their schedules to accommodate the cleansing process and allow for more rest time, which is advisable, though not a requirement.

During this cleanse, you *might* exhibit symptoms such as nausea, headache, aching liver, grouchiness, low energy, hot flashes, anger, depression, high energy, discontent, agitation, and irritability. Don't be alarmed — these are all common cleansing reactions as not only physical toxins clear out, but also emotional ones. The liver stores our passions and our frustrations. Suppressed emotions may be released, so give yourself permission to express them by shouting, screaming, punching a pillow, crying, or whatever you need to do in a *safe and private way* (instead of inappropriately venting on your loved ones). The beauty of the cleansing process is that when stored emotions are safely released, you're left with a greater capacity to embrace life in the present and express the more productive nature of passion. It is also fine to have no overt reactions, since this varies for each person — trust that cleansing is happening!

Day 1: Upon rising, drink 8 ounces of purified water. Follow this with the liver-flush drink previously described. Fifteen minutes after drinking this wonderful concoction, follow it with *2 cups* of *Detoxification Decoction* and *40–60 drops* (1 teaspoon) of *Liver-Gallbladder Tincture* (recipes below). For breakfast you may drink fresh fruit juices (always dilute juices with one-third part water), fruit smoothies with super-foods, fresh, in-season fruits, and soaked nuts. Stop all fruit consumption one hour before lunch.

For lunch, take *40–60 more drops of tincture with one cup of detoxification decoction*, plus diluted fresh vegetable juices, *any* raw vegetables (includes avocado) alone or in salad, sprouts, seeds, and potassium broth (see day 3). You can make your own dressing for the salad using olive oil, herbs, garlic, ginger, lemon, raw tahini, and apple cider vinegar, etc. Afternoon snacks and dinner can be raw vegetables (more salad!), vegetable juices, sprouts, potassium broth, and herb teas. Take another *40–60 drops of tincture with one more cup of detoxification decoction*. Stop consuming vegetables by 8:00 P.M.

In the evening, at least one hour after you've stopped ingesting vegetables, you may consume fruits and their juices if needed. Then take the *last dose of tincture*. Be sure to drink four quarts of spring or distilled water throughout the day.

Day 2: Repeat as for day 1!

Day 3: Start the day with water, the flush, the decoction, and the tincture, but this time, eat no solid food, only diluted fruit juices in the morning. From noon until 8 P.M. you may have diluted vegetable juices and potassium broth.

 ## Potassium Broth

Fill a large pot with 25 percent chopped organic potatoes, 25 percent chopped organic onions and garlic, 25 percent chopped organic carrots and beets, and 25 percent chopped celery and dark, leafy greens such as beet tops, plus any herbs or sea vegetables desired. Cover with purified water, bring to a boil, then simmer, very low, for 2 hours; strain, and drink only the broth — compost the peelings.

It's easiest to make a large batch of broth that will last two to three days in the refrigerator. Heat the broth to serve, adding cayenne pepper and a little olive oil, wheat germ oil, or flaxseed oil to taste — yum! This broth will flush your system of unwanted salts and acids while providing a concentrated amount of vitamins and minerals.

Be sure to get in your *40 – 60 drops of tincture and one cup of detoxification decoction four times a day*. In the late evening, it's back to diluted fruit juices; if your bowels tend to be sluggish, warm prune juice before going to bed is a good idea.

Days 4 and 5: (day 5 is for a seven-day cleanse) are the same as day 3. Consume *at least* four quarts of water per day (about 1 cup every hour). If you get hungry, *drink more!*

Day 5 or 6: Today you break your juice fast. Make this day the same as day 1 by starting with water, the flush, the decoction and tincture, and diluted fruit juices. Slowly begin eating fresh fruit, chew thoroughly, and eat only until satisfied, *not full.* For lunch and dinner you may have small vegetable salads, vegetable juices, and potassium broth, and in the evening a fruit smoothie, fruit salad, or juices. If you're intolerant of fruit sugars, simply continue with raw vegetables/juices and potassium broth into the evening. Be sure to take *40 – 60 drops of tincture and one cup of decoction four times per day* — plus lots of water!

Day 7: The same as day 6. If you're on the five-day cleanse, you'll do two days of liquids only and end on the fifth day, or repeat day five for a six-day version.

To end your cleanse, start your day the same as day 1 and then *ease* your way into the Revitalizing Diet. Begin by eating lightly and more frequently, and *continue drinking plenty of water.* A common mistake is for people to drastically cut their fluid intake once they're eating solid, and often drier, foods again, which typically results in intestinal unhappiness! Please note that if you weigh less than one hundred pounds, you should reduce the tincture and decoction dosages accordingly (see appendix). If you liver cleanse in very cold weather and you find too much raw food depleting, then add finely grated raw foods to lightly steamed vegetables and slow-cooked grains. This program can be done on a one-week-on, one-week-off basis for up to three weeks of cleansing, until you feel that deep-seated imbalances have shifted.

Detoxification Decoction

2 parts each: dandelion root, burdock root, pau d'arco bark, and knotweed — also called fo-ti or He Shou Wu (*Polygonum multiflorum*)

1 part each: echinacea root, ginger root, licorice root, cinnamon bark, sarsaparilla, uva ursi leaf (*Arctostaphylos uva ursi*), and horsetail

½ part each: carob pod (or half of this portion of carob powder), whole clove, fennel seed, juniper berry, and orange peel

¼ part each: black peppercorns and chaparral — or as close to this combination as you can get

*If you can only find an herb in tincture, simply add a few drops of the tincture to your pot of herbs. If your bowels are sluggish, add **½ part** of cascara sagrada bark.*

Liver-Gallbladder Tincture

3 parts milk thistle seed

1 part each: dandelion root and leaf, Oregon grape root, barberry root bark, artichoke leaf, wormwood, Turkey rhubarb, and aniseed

½ part gentian root

Parasites like to hang out in the liver as well. This tincture contain anti-parasitic herbs, but if you feel you need something stronger, add one part neem seed or take Para-gone! tincture (chapter one).

Other activities to include while on liver cleansing:

1. Skin brushing and alternating hot and cold showers to aid the skin in releasing toxins (always end showers with cool water). Saunas and massages are also stimulating.

2. Taking a warm bath in the evening with Epsom and sea salts and essential oils (ginger, rosemary, coriander, and lemon grass or Melissa / lemon balm are recommended).

3. A minimum of twenty minutes of cardiovascular exercise daily.

4. Deep belly breathing or meditation each morning and evening for ten to fifteen minutes.

5. Put a castor-oil pack over your liver if you feel discomfort. This is essentially a compress made by saturating a cloth with warm castor oil, placing it over the liver, and covering it with cellophane or plastic, then a towel, and finally a hot-water bottle or electric heating pad.

6. Spending time in nature, especially among trees, is nourishing for your liver!

I am the Source, I dream the dreams, I am the light,
Creation lives in me, Creation lives in me...

— a nice chant while cleansing

While our liver regulates the flow of life energy and blood in our body, this flow is easily disrupted by excessive or negative emotions, or over-stimulation (as with alcohol, drugs, caffeine, or an excess of hot spices). The liver also harmonizes digestion as well as influencing the integrity of joints, ligaments, tendons, nails, and muscular pain. While dietary factors are key in liver function, so are temperature (hot weather provokes our liver), over-activity without rest, overwork, and "hot" emotions such as anger and frustration toward others that remain unexpressed or unresolved. Being unafraid to assert yourself, but doing so with consideration for others, makes a happy liver! So does staying out of toxic environments, including toxic relationships.

Chemical exposure can make you sick! It's very important to keep away from chemical cleansers, paints, gases, and perfumes while cleansing your liver, since it is *releasing toxins it might normally hold.* It is possible to experience toxic shock if exposed to strong chemicals while the liver is flushing. Foods such as artichokes, olives, and bitter greens are particularly nourishing, and ginger will reduce nausea due to chemical exposure. Homeopathic detoxification remedies (such as Body Pure by BHI — see source list), flower remedies, castor-oil packs on the liver, and the amino-acid supplement NAC (N-Acetyl Cysteine) can help reduce symptoms of nausea and headache.

The Mega-Gallbladder-Liver Purge

Blood-cleansing organs and areas such as the bowel and liver are highly subject to parasites. Blood parasites can settle in the liver and attach to liver stones. For some organisms, such as liver flukes, the liver is part of their life cycle. The liver has an active immune system and is surrounded by lymphatic vessels that help remove debris, but if blood flow through the liver becomes congested, or the liver is severely compromised by heavy toxic load or necrosis (death of liver cells), it can no longer rid itself of parasites, bacteria, and viruses.

The following mega-purge is extremely effective but must be executed with great care, preferably with professional guidance. *Never* do this without first doing a thorough bowel cleansing (ideally, using a colonic board the day before) and a basic liver cleanse! This flush will release liver stones, gall stones and parasites, but will be most useful if repeated every two to four weeks until there are very few stones (fewer than fifty) being eliminated. It's more comfortable and more efficient if you can get on a colonic board the morning after the flush to release the stones; otherwise, you'll want to be close to a toilet for the first half of the day! The mega-gallbladder-liver purge goes as follows:

Two Days Before

Eat only soft foods, smoothies, pureed soups, juices — in essence baby food. Don't consume the skins of fruits and vegetables, do not eat seeded berries, husks of grains and eat no animal products. Take one bowel capsule with your dinner each evening and 2 teaspoons liquid clay plus 2 teaspoons *powdered* psyllium husk in ten ounces of water one hour before bed. *Don't forget to drink a gallon of water each day!* On the day before the flush, clean out the colon with a gravity-fed herbal flush if possible (consult a trained colon therapist as necessary).

Day of Purge

All eating and drinking must end by 2 P.M. Eat only soft foods, but absolute-ly *no fat!* Many fruits and vegetables have fat (bananas, avocados, legumes, seeds and nuts, coconut, garlic, and onion, etc.). Just stick to what *is* essen-tially fat-free: all squashes, potatoes and yams (no skins), steamed broccoli or cauliflower, applesauce, vegetable juices, green grasses (spirulina, barley, algae), carrot juice — *keep it simple — do not take any supplements or herbal formulas.* Drink as much of one gallon water as possible.

At 2 p.m.: *Stop all intake of foods and fluids.* The reason for this is to allow the liver and gallbladder to rest (fats and fluids activate them). The liver will actually deflate and "sleep." If at any time you feel tired, headachy, nauseated, or irritable, remember to slow down, get fresh air, rest as needed, and help yourself by misting essential oils such as lemon, grapefruit, rosemary, gin-ger, or lavender. Nurture your body by receiving some energy work or light bodywork and loving yourself.

At 6 p.m.: Drink 1 tablespoon of Epsom salts in ¾ cup water; follow this with a dot of honey on your tongue to remove the bitter aftertaste. You have to heat the water first to get the salts to dissolve, then let it cool, so best to prepare this half an hour ahead of time. The Epsom salts will pull water into your bowel and cause it to evacuate its contents over the next hour.

At 8 p.m.: Relish another glass of Epsom-salts water as above. During the next two hours, try to eliminate and urinate as much as possible; massaging your lower belly helps.

At 9:30 p.m.: Start preparing for bed, and make one more dose of Epsom-salts water for use later, then make the following bedtime cocktail:

½ cup strained juice of one refrigerated (cool) grapefruit, preferably pink; one-half cup of *extra-light* olive oil (nearly clear in color).

Put in a jar, close the lid, and take it to your bedside.

At 10 p.m.: Get cozy, sit in bed, shake the grapefruit cocktail vigorously, and drink it down — it's the best-tasting drink you can imagine after Epsom salts! Turn off your bedside light or candle, lie on your *left* side, and *do not* *move* for at least thirty minutes, preferably one hour, and sail into dreamland. You might feel your liver expand and contract as though it were letting out a big sigh of relief as the oil and sour juice instantly activate it, causing it to release bile, stones, and any other lingering items into the gallbladder, which squeezes debris into the intestines to be eliminated out the bowel. After an hour, if your bowel is activated, get up to eliminate, but usually, hours pass before there is any such urgency. Anytime *after* 3 A.M., you may have one more dose of Epsom-salt water, which will insure evacuation of stones and debris that by this time have made it into the large intestine. Do not drink any water until two hours after your last Epsom dose. If you're getting on a colonic board for a full flush in the morning, you may omit this last dose of salts.

The next morning: If you aren't using a colonic board, simply stay within easy reach of a toilet for the first half of the day, as you'll be eliminating in increments.

Be sure to take a look at what you are eliminating! Liver stones float on the surface of the water and come in all shades of amber from cream to deep orange. They are shaped the way they were wedged in the blood vessel, and larger ones may sport the tails of parasites. Gallstones also float, are normally green and round, and may also have parasites attached to them.

The morning after the flush, begin drinking water again, one gallon a day, while introducing soft foods; stay on soft foods for two more days, taking two teaspoons of liquid clay and two teaspoons of powdered psyllium husk in water each evening. Follow up with anti-parasitic herbs and acidophilus capsules, morning and evenings, for seven to ten days.

Typically, doing this mega-purge the first time results in many lentil-sized stones, but as you repeat the procedure, larger stones and more parasites, if there are any, will be released. Other things you might notice are a sticky, white, stringy film of cholesterol floating near the surface, or yellow foam from bile salts, or mucus and waste from the bowel. Either way, say good riddance and give yourself and your liver a big hug!

Though the mega-purge sounds drastic, it's less so than having one's gallbladder removed, or suffering serious liver disease. Contrary to popular belief, the gallbladder is a necessary organ. Once it is removed, the concentrated flow of bile delivered into the small intestine to help digest and absorb fat, is replaced by a more continuous, less concentrated drip directly from the liver. This often results in gastrointestinal complaints such as bloating, gas, diarrhea, and pain in the upper abdomen. To mitigate these effects, one must then be very careful about eating fats. Digestive enzymes are usually needed before each meal to compensate. Removal of organs should always be considered a last option, although such extreme measures may be warranted. Preventive care, along with listening and responding to early warning signs is far less extreme and more often leads to authentic healing.

Bitter herbs or herbal tonics, which are a European tradition, can be taken just before and / or just after main meals to help activate the liver and stimulate bile production. Taking bitters consistently in the correct dosage for one's constitution will prevent buildup of stones. If you experience pain or discomfort of the liver / gallbladder, which can happen during cleansing or otherwise, lie down with a warm castor-oil pack over the area and rest. Homeopathic Nux vomica can help. If you're experiencing a gallbladder attack — sharp pain and nausea caused by a stone becoming stuck in the bile duct — stop all food and drink, lie down with a castor-oil pack, and suck on a piece of lemon or ginger to counter nausea. Once symptoms subside, gently begin with the basic liver flush and consume only liquids. Prepare the Bye-bye Bile decoction below, adding to it ½ part crampbark. If symptoms persist, with vomiting, *do not hesitate — seek professional help immediately!*

Help for Common Ailments

Jaundice

Jaundice shows as a yellowing of the skin and the whites of the eyes, and indicates congestion within the liver that leads to a buildup of bile pigment (bilirubin) in the blood. It can be a symptom of obstruction of the bile duct (usually a gallstone), or disease of the liver due to infection, hepatitis, alcoholism, poisons, or anorexia, in which there is an excessive destruction of red blood cells. Jaundice in newborns is caused by the destruction of excess hemoglobin in red blood cells, and usually disappears spontaneously. The underlying cause of jaundice must be addressed. Eating bitter and sour foods and herbs can begin to release excess bile into the bowel where it is eliminated. Drink one-half cup of the following decoction every two hours while symptoms last.

Bye-bye Bile

1 part each: fringe tree bark, dandelion root, Oregon grape root, and marshmallow root

½ part each: wild yam and fennel or anise seed

Prepare as a decoction and drink one-half cup at a time.

Hepatitis

Hepatitis is inflammation of the liver, with accompanying liver cell damage or death. Hepatitis is characterized by jaundice, lack of appetite, abdominal discomfort, nausea, vomiting, enlarged liver, abnormal function of the liver, and dark urine. It is often caused by bacterial or viral infection, or infestation with parasites, but can also be caused by alcohol, drugs, toxins, transfusions of incompatible or infected blood, or as a complication of another disease such as infectious mononucleosis. There are several types of hepatitis viruses, and hepatitis can be acute or chronic.

The most common acute form, hepatitis E (Hep E) is brought on by bacterial infection, usually in contaminated food. Addressing the problem immediately, during the acute stage (nausea and vomiting), is most important; for this, tincture of neem seed is very effective. Take one teaspoon three times a day for three days, then one teaspoon twice a day for two days. Most important, remain hydrated by drinking electrolyte solutions and replenishing the body with potassium broth, super-greens (wheat, barley, spirulina, and kamut grasses), and sea vegetables. Once diarrhea and nausea have stopped, make soups with shiitake mushroom, burdock root, ginger, turmeric, barley, nettle, celery, root vegetables, and legumes (lentils, mung beans, or aduki beans). Prepare Detoxification Decoction to cleanse the blood, and drink three cups a day for one week. Oil of oregano or oregano-leaf tincture and / or olive leaf can be taken for a time afterward to continue warding off pathogens. Turmeric, eleuthero (Eleutherococcus senticosus), milk thistle, and schizandra berry are excellent for long-term care, as well as fresh-pressed carrot-parsley-ginger juice.

Viral hepatitis A (Hep A) is caused by a virus present in the feces of infected people, and is transmitted through food and infected water. Sometimes referred to as traveler's hepatitis, it is similar to and can be treated as acute hepatitis, described above, except symptoms may appear later as flu-like illness with jaundice.

Viral hepatitis B (Hep B) is present in blood and other body fluids of infected people; it is spread through sexual contact or infected blood, or passed on to infants while in the womb. Hep B can be asymptomatic or show itself as abdominal pain, jaundice, nausea, general malaise, vomiting, or joint pain. This virus can persist for years, becoming chronic and causing intense inflammation and destruction of liver cells. Scar tissue can form and lead to cirrhosis of the liver.

Viral Hepatitis C (Hep C), is usually passed on by contaminated blood or hypodermic needles; however up to 40 percent of all cases appear from "unknown causes." Beginning to reach epidemic proportions, Hepatitis C typically results in chronic liver disease and deterioration of the organ; the virus can, however, go into remission.

Any chronic hepatitis can also result from an autoimmune reaction, a reaction to medication, or, more rarely, a metabolic disorder. Treatment of chronic hepatitis should include boosting the immune system, preventing cell death with antiviral herbs (e.g., St. John's wort, thuja, olive leaf, ligustrum (Ligustrum lucidum), reishi, maitake (Grifola frondosa), shiitake, and other medicinal mushrooms, enhancing liver regeneration (using milk thistle and antioxidants), increasing bile flow and elimination of wastes, and addressing addictions. To relieve liver inflammation, remove stressors such as alcohol, red meat dairy products, spicy, warming foods such as garlic, cayenne, pepper, and curries, and cooking with oil. Adopt a light diet built on greens (lightly steamed), whole grains, and legumes. Include steamed nettles and other bitter greens such as dandelion leaf, and soaked almonds, flaxseed, and walnuts, and eat plenty of super-foods. It's best to let food cool to nearly room temperature before eating. The major herbs for hepatitis and cirrhosis of the liver are milk thistle and mugwort (or other *Artemisia* spp.), taken in concentrated extract form as tablets, powder, or alcohol-free tincture. Other potent herbs are fringe tree, bulpleurum, rosemary, turmeric, olive, eat artichoke leaf, grape leaf (*Vitis vinifera*), dandelion root, Oregon grape, oregano, gentian, and rhodiola rhizome (*Rhodiola rosea*). Use castor-oil packs to soothe the liver, and arrange to receive bodywork, acupuncture, or acupressure treatment whenever possible, while seeking professional guidance.

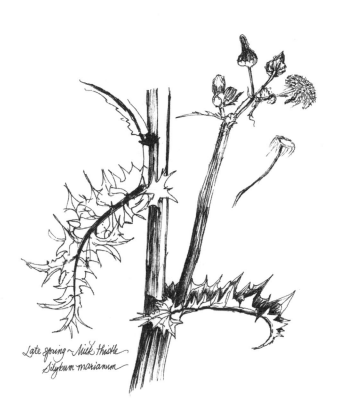

Late spring ~ Milk thistle
Silybum marianum

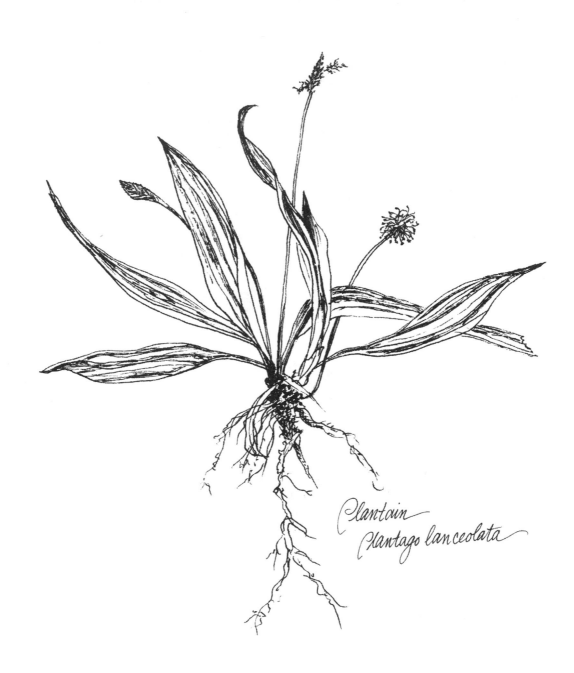

Plantain
Plantago lanceolata

Chapter Four

The Circulatory System:
Heart, Vessels, Bones, and Skin

A heart full of love always has something to give.
Anonymous

L ike the sap of a tree, a fluid travels through us, delivering oxygen, nutrients, antioxidants, hormone messengers, antibodies, and water to all our tissues, while simultaneously carrying away carbon dioxide and other waste products. This protein-rich fluid of life-force energy is blood, red as the molten center of the earth and holding our inner fire. Our circulatory system is a system of commerce and exchange; its activity keeps our body's economy enriched. It is responsible for transporting the goods we need to stay alive, and wherever it flows freely, there is vibrant energy, rejuvenation, and renewal. When blood flow is inhibited, everything slows down; vessels becomes overcrowded, sticky, blocked, inefficient, and unable to deliver essential nutrients. The vitality of our circulatory system is fundamental to life and to the connection and integration of all parts of our body.

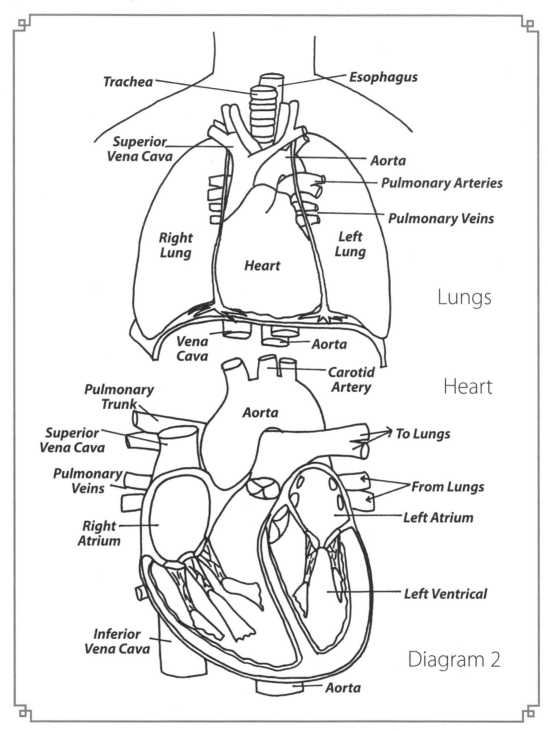

Trachea

Esophagus

Superior Vena Cava

Aorta

Pulmonary Arteries

Pulmonary Veins

Right Lung

Left Lung

Heart

Lungs

Vena Cava

Aorta

Carotid Artery

Heart

Pulmonary Trunk

Aorta

Superior Vena Cava

To Lungs

Pulmonary Veins

From Lungs

Right Atrium

Left Atrium

Left Ventrical

Inferior Vena Cava

Diagram 2

Aorta

The circulatory system is composed of the heart, the components of blood (red and white blood cells, salts, water, oxygen, and other nutrients), arteries, veins, and capillaries. It can be divided into two major parts: *systemic circulation,* which supplies blood to your entire body except the lungs; and *pulmonary circulation,* whereby blood is re-oxygenated by cycling through the lungs. Blood is a connective tissue, as are cartilage, ligaments, skin, and bone; like all connective tissues, blood has the ability to build and repair itself. Building and repairing of connective tissue relies on a steady flow of nutrients that the river of blood provides. If blood flow stagnates, there is pain or numbness, coldness and stiffness, swelling and bruising. When this continues over time, illness, disease, and loss of function occur. Gangrene is the most severe form of blood stagnation. Our overall health depends on the steady flow of this life-giving river, and the source of its movement is our heart.

The Heart

Your heart is a self-contained muscle that receives deoxygenated blood from veins and pumps re-oxygenated blood into arteries. Its own set of vessels (coronary arteries and veins) nourish and sustain it, and, like all muscle tissue, it has the capacity to strengthen, weaken, become more elastic or static, and recover from trauma or damage. It is the main station linking the systemic and pulmonary circulation systems. In Oriental healing traditions, the heart is said to house the spirit or "*Shen,*" which presides over all body functions with awareness and wisdom. In Western healing traditions, the heart is said to be the seat of love and understanding, and the key to emotional well-being. Many spiritual traditions acknowledge the heart as a unique expression of the confluence of spirit and matter, or the interconnectedness between our perceptions of the internal versus external environment. Indeed, our breath or *prana* (spirit we inhale) is processed by the pulmonary system to feed the matter of our bodies.

Our heart is directly influenced, both energetically and physiologically, by the state of our small intestine, which separates and sorts out substances entering the blood, thereby purifying the blood of negative influences and protecting the heart. Symptoms like indigestion (heartburn) result when this sorting process is not complete. Our heart can feel pressured when the bowel — particularly the transverse colon and splenic flexure — is filled with waste material and pushes up on the diaphragm and chest to put pressure on the pericardium, the protective sac encasing the heart. Our heart is also influenced by the health of our kidneys, since fluid retention raises blood pressure and thus pressure on the heart.

The pulmonary circulatory system moves oxygen-poor blood, collected from our body by the veins, into the largest vein (vena cava), which empties into the right side of our heart (see diagram 2, page 76). It is pumped from the right ventricle into the main pulmonary vein, which flows to the lungs. Here the deoxygenated blood moves into smaller and smaller vessels until it reaches the capillary beds in the lung sacs called alveoli. Like a relay team, venous capillaries pass on waste products (CO_2 and various gases), which are released as you exhale, and catch fresh oxygen (O_2) from arterial capillaries in the lungs to pass back to your heart. This refreshed, bright red blood flows back into the left side of your heart and is pumped into the aorta to begin its journey through your entire systemic circulatory system. It is a highly efficient cycle as long as we keep moving and breathing, since venous flow is against gravity and needs our assistance.

The coronary arteries and veins that lace the outside of our heart have their own miniature version of this process as waste from muscle activity is replaced with oxygen-rich blood that feeds the heart muscle itself. Coronary vessels are subject to the same pampering, or abuse, as your general circulation. Myocardial infarction is a stoppage of blood flow in the coronary vessels. Cardiovascular disease accounts for more deaths in the USA than any other cause of death, including cancer and AIDS. This includes heart attacks, strokes, and CVD (congestive heart failure), of which fewer than 20 percent are due to genetic malfunction. The remaining 80 percent of deaths are attributed to dietary habits, stress, viruses, side effects from pharmaceutical drugs, and lifestyle, which can also include the cumulative effects of exposure to electromagnetic radiation.

Care of our heart requires a peaceful state of mind and a diet rich in fresh fruits, vegetables, and grains. Bitter foods are very supportive to both the heart and small intestine, as are red, black, or blue fruits and vegetables. Onions, leeks, and garlic are master cleansers, while whole organic grains of wheat (bulgur or cracked wheat, wheat germ, wheat grass) help cool and clear the blood, easing any inflammation. Inflammation, a big culprit in heart disease, is primarily caused by eating high amounts of sugar, and saturated, cooked, or rancid fats — all detrimental to the circulatory system because they speed up the oxidation (decay) process of cells and cause blood platelets to stick, thus increasing tissue demands for more oxygen. You can reduce this deterioration process by avoiding meat, cheese, cream, chips, cakes, cookies, pastries, mayonnaise, oil-based granola, roasted nuts, and "snack foods." *Always read labels carefully* and *run* from those that say hydrogenated or fractionated oil (such as in margarine, candies, and many crackers and chips). Stick to cold-pressed extra-virgin olive oil, and store other unsaturated oils or nut butters in the refrigerator. Oils from fish, flax, coconut, macadamia nut, black currant, evening primrose, and borage contain omega-3 fatty acids that actually *reduce* inflammation and cholesterol levels.

Cholesterol, a vital part of cell-membrane structure, is needed for bile formation, hormone production, and vitamin D synthesis. Our bodies produce much of the cholesterol we need in our liver. Excess dietary cholesterol is held in the liver and deposited on artery walls. Salt increases blood pressure by constricting vessels, and is far too prevalent in commercial cooking and household recipes. Using plenty of herbs and spices usually negates the need for salt, but good alternatives to table salt are sea vegetables, potassium salt, or Bragg Liquid Aminos (an unfermented soy product). Alcohol increases strain on the circulation and the heart by forceful dilation of blood vessels, which can cause capillaries in our skin to burst.

Do not smoke. Smoking accounts for the highest risk in heart failure. Nicotine also dilates capillaries, causing them to burst, usually on the face and fingers. Likewise, stimulants like caffeine put undue stress on our heart by upsetting normal electrolyte balance and disturbing tissue fluids (thus pressure). Stimulants also mimic the fight-or-flight stress response that raises vascular pressure, raises blood sugar, and reduces blood flow to our organs.

Foods high in salicylate help keep blood platelets from becoming sticky and clumping together. These include lemons, oranges, almonds, grapefruits, peaches, prunes, figs, rhubarb, cherries, melons / cucumbers, nectarines, plums / prunes, persimmons, currants, raisins, raw tomatoes, apples, and pineapple; always eat the skins when possible. Meadowsweet and white willow bark are herbs especially rich in salicylate. Pure aspirin is acetylsalicylic acid, often recommended for heart patients. Unfortunately, aspirin is extremely toxic to the liver, particularly the buffered varieties, due to petrochemical residues, and is therefore counterproductive to health over the long term.

Considering how many foods in nature readily provide this acid, it's far wiser to eat a nutritious diet, especially because whole plants provide additional substances to aid results. For example, the vitamin C in all the fruits listed above is a strong antioxidant that improves elasticity of veins. The inner skins of citrus are an excellent source of bioflavonoids (vitamin P) and rutin, which strengthen and tone vessel walls. Eucalyptus-leaf tea and buckwheat sprouts are rich sources of rutin to include in your diet as well.

Don't forget a daily intake and outpouring of love and joyous expression! *Following your heart* is still one of the best treatments you can give yourself. Here's a healthy heart tonic:

Healthy Heart Tincture

3 parts each: hawthorn leaf and berry (*Crataegus oxycantha*)

2 parts motherwort (*Leonuris cardiaca*) **leaf**

1 part each: gingko (*Gingko biloba*) and olive leaf

½ part each: rosemary, cayenne pepper, and lobelia

This can be made into a tincture or tea (using fresh hawthorn berries) and taken daily to tone and calm the heart.

To support and strengthen your heart, use herbs such as aloe leaf, borage leaf and flower (*Borago officinalis*), hawthorn berry leaf and flower, figwort, and bean pods — yes, beans are good for the heart! Herbs that help regulate our heart muscle include night-blooming cereus cactus (*Salenicereus grandiflorus*), cayenne pepper, lobelia, blue vervain, linden flower, also called lime blossom (*Tilia europaea*), passionflower (*Passiflora incarnata*), and motherwort (*Leonorus cardiaca*). Herbs such as garlic, gingko, elecampane, and olive leaf have high antioxidant value and provide general assistance by supporting the entire pulmonary system. Try the following tea for nurturing this beloved muscle.

Heart-ease Tea

2 parts each: hawthorn leaf and flower, linden blossom, and lemon balm (*Melissa officinalis*)

1 part each: rose petals, rose hips, and red raspberry leaf

Sip two to three cups per day

A heart attack (also called a coronary) is tissue death of an area of the heart muscle caused by interrupted blood supply due to blockage of coronary arteries. The blockage is usually a blood clot within an artery previously narrowed by atherosclerosis (a form of arteriosclerosis). Maintaining a whole-foods diet, doing daily aerobic exercise (not to the point of exhaustion), and addressing anxiety and stress (disturbances of the spirit), will reduce the risk of heart attack. Grief over love lost is a significant factor in heart disease; therefore it's important to confront issues that have "broken your heart." Herbal formulas that contain hawthorn berry, such as Healthy Heart Tonic, plus any appropriate *nervines* (see chapter eight), can be taken to protect the heart. In the event of heart attack or stroke, a few droppers full of *emergency tincture* while waiting for emergency care may sustain a person until medical help arrives. If you are having a heart attack and are alone, taking emergency tincture, plus trying to cough repeatedly, which uses the diaphragm to stimulate the heart muscle, may save your life.

Emergency Tincture

Combine equal parts cayenne tincture (any hot chili pepper — the hotter the better) and tincture of lobelia

12 drops of Bach flower rescue remedy (Five Flower Remedy) for a one-ounce bottle

Fill a half-ounce bottle (labeled clearly) and carry with you.

In recovering from a heart attack, lifestyle changes along with bodywork and acupuncture are necessary. Taking GLA (*Gamma Linolenic Acid*) in the form of oil of borage, primrose, or black currant seed, will affect prostaglandin metabolism to prevent sticky platelets and inflammation of the heart muscle. High blood sugar causes inflammation and oxidation of heart muscle. Eliminating sugar and high-starch foods will mitigate this. Other herbs that effectively address inflammation of the heart muscle are turmeric, ginger, holy basil / tulsi, Baikal or Chinese skullcap (*Scutellaria baicalensis*), dandelion, wheatgrass, rosemary, oregano, feverfew (*Tanacetum parthenium*) and hops.

Essential Fatty Acids

Essential fatty acids (omega 3 and 6) should make up at least one-third of the oils in your diet. Omega-6 fatty acids are prevalent in many vegetables, nuts, and seeds in the form of *linoleic acid* (LA), and are converted in our bodies to *gamma linolenic acid* (GLA) and *arachidonic acid* (AA). Omega-3 oils, found in some nuts and seeds (especially walnuts, macadamia nuts, coconut, and flax), include *alpha linolenic acid* (ALA) whose derivatives, *eicosapentaenoic acid* (EPA) and *docosahexaenoic acid* (DHA), are produced in our bodies. EPA is especially supportive to the vascular system, and DHA is restorative to the nervous system and brain. All essential fatty acids are precursors to various prostaglandins that promote skin integrity, joint lubrication, regulate blood pressure, balance hormone production, lower triglyceride levels, regulate immune function, manage inflammation in the body, and protect cell membranes, especially in the brain. Essential fatty acids can be ingested via soaked nuts and seeds, nut butters such as raw sesame tahini or almond butter, ground flaxseed, wheat germ, and coconut, or supplemental oils of borage seed, evening primrose seed, black currant seed, hemp seed, macadamia nut, pumpkinseed, flaxseed, and walnut.

Regulation of inflammation is part of the immune response, and balance is the key. While GLA found in plant foods is a strong anti-inflammatory, AA is more prevalent in animal fats and is a precursor to prostaglandins that increase inflammation. The omega-3 oils are also abundant in wild-caught cold-water fish, such as salmon, herring, cod, and sardines. Marine algae are the primary sources of omega-3 oils in the food chain; fish feed on the algae, absorb the ALA, and convert it to DHA and EPA in their tissues, making it readily available.

Two to three 4-ounce servings of cold-water fish per week provide a rich, easily assimilated helping of omega-3 oils, and contain other supportive proteins especially important for those whose health is severely compromised. Be responsible about fish consumption: remember that all fish carry various loads of heavy metals, and the oceans today are over-fished. The richest land source of omega-3 oils is flaxseed, which can be ground and sprinkled on food or added to smoothies, or you can take the oil — up to two tablespoons a day, or in capsules, five to six days a week.

Other Connective Tissues

Ligaments, tendons, and cartilage are made up of collagen fibers forming an elastic matrix of cells that have the ability to build and repair tissue. They provide us bounce and mobility as long as they are well nourished and given the freedom to find their own movement.

Antagonistic to the support of the skeletal is repetitive movement, which limits the use and blood flow to a particular area. Stretching and natural movement, particularly before and after repetitive activities, is the best way to prevent problems! Foods and herbs that nourish the bloodstream in general also nourish these tissues. Herbs specific to the liver will help relieve swelling and pain due to blood stagnation. Antioxidants, necessary weight loss, water therapy, yoga, and massage, all of which stimulate collagen production, can also heal connective tissue.

An herbal poultice combination such as hops, St. John's wort, arnica (*Arnica montana*), and ginger can be applied directly to the area to relieve aching. Herbs taken internally that relax connective tissue and muscles include gotu-kola (*Hydrocotyle asiatica*), sweet marjoram (*Origanum majorana*), kava kava (*Piper methysticum*), lobelia, lemon balm, lavender, cramp bark, skunk cabbage root, birch bark, and wild yam. Topically applied liniments made from essential oils will penetrate deeply into tissues. Look for those containing one or more of the following: wintergreen (*Gaultheria procumbens*), cayenne, peppermint, oregano, camphor (*Cinnamomum camphora*), arnica, St. John's wort, calendula, ginger, clove, basil, all marjorams, birch, or mustard. Some of these herbs, like mustard and cayenne, serve as rubefacients — herbs that draw toxins from the site of injury or swelling to the surface of the skin by stimulating topical circulation. Herbs that promote tissue regeneration are called vulneraries. It's helpful to complement external application with internal use. Effective vulneraries that can be used internally and externally are plantain leaf, selfheal flower spike (*Prunella vulgaris*), comfrey leaf, boneset (*Eupatorium perfoliatum*), St. John's wort, grapevine, gotu-kola, yarrow (*Achillea millefolium*), and aloe vera leaf.

Ligaments are bands or sheets of connective tissue linking two or more bones or cartilage structures. They also serve as support for muscles and fascia (layers of tissue that cover muscle). When ligaments are twisted or torn, they heal best with ice-cold compresses for the first twenty-four hours, then warm, damp heat and water therapy. Massage with essential oils (oregano, marjoram, rosemary, black pepper), gentle movement therapy, and do strengthening exercises for surrounding (supporting) muscle. Natural plant sulfur in the supplemental powder MSM (methyl sulfonyl methane) will help speed tissue repair, along with a nutrient-rich diet including fresh vegetable juices and sea minerals. Homeopathic *Ruta graveolens* or *Bellis perennis* can also be taken.

Tendons are fibrous bands or cords that are part of the muscle and connect the fleshy, contractile portion of it with bone. When they are over-stretched or inflamed, tendons prefer ice-cold compresses, alternating hot and cold packs, rest, and deep massage or acupressure at the points of muscle attachment. Topically applied liniments that are cooling, such as wintergreen, peppermint, eucalyptus, or camphor, are soothing. Homeopathic *Apis* and *Ledum* can be helpful.

Cartilage is connective tissue without blood vessels. Found primarily in the joints, the walls of the chest, and in tubular structures (trachea, larynx, air passages, ear canals), cartilage comprises most of the skeleton in early fetal life before it is slowly replaced by bone. Due to its lack of blood vessels, it's not able to repair easily; in fact, it is dependent on the strength and circulation of surrounding tissues in general, and the health of the blood, lymph, and liver in particular. Therefore herbs, foods, and therapies that are building for all connective tissues can be applied in cases of cartilage damage.

Bones

Bones hold our essence and are linked to the vitality of our kidneys. Marrow, the living center of bone, is the source of our red blood cells and primary immune cells. The bone marrow feeds our blood as the blood feeds the marrow, in the same way we give to our community as our community supports us. Psychologically, it's about giving and receiving support. Bones both support and are supported by muscles, tendons, and ligaments.

Bones are our mineral bank account—don't let the balance drop down too far! Our bodies are about 4 percent mineral by weight (whereas vitamins comprise 1 percent) and calcium and phosphorus account for 75 percent of that. Ninety-nine percent of all calcium in our bodies, along with 70 percent of all magnesium, is stored in our bones and teeth. Storage of minerals in bone is your special savings account, which you draw from in pregnancy or while recovering from injury or illness. Minerals, particularly calcium, are also spent to alkalize (increase the pH of) your blood should it become too acidic. Foods and beverages such as sodas, coffee, black tea, alcohol, red meat, sugar, refined packaged foods, acidic drinking water, and some pharmaceutical drugs, cause our blood to shift to an acid condition. Repetitive stress, cold weather, heavy-metal poisoning, low hormone levels, and fevers also use up blood minerals; unless they are replaced immediately, the loss can lead to an acid condition.

Our bodies quickly respond to such changes in blood acidity by drawing from our bone bank. Like any account, if you replace the funds you use, a balance is kept, but if you become overdrawn, you create an impoverished mineral condition, which can eventually lead to *osteoporosis* (tiny holes in the bones). If you're building or repairing tissue, eating lots of sweets, or are under constant stress, for example, you must support your body with needed calcium, magnesium, phosphorus, and trace minerals (boron, zinc, manganese, and copper). Include in your diet herbs such as sea vegetables, nettle, red raspberry leaf, alfalfa, and other grasses. High-calcium tea (see common ailments, this chapter) and potassium broth (see appendix) are a good start. Low stomach acid will reduce the absorption of minerals from your diet, so attend to stomach acid if it needs balancing. Purifying and alkalizing your blood, and fortifying it with minerals, along with regular weight-bearing exercise, will build strong bones.

Teeth

Teeth are part of the skeletal system, and, in fact, move with spinal changes. They also strengthen or weaken in accordance with the overall state of our bones. Therefore, any bone-building herbs assist the teeth greatly, especially those high in calcium, magnesium, vitamin D, and phosphorus. Inadequate dental hygiene can contribute to inflamed arteries and blood clots, leading to cardiovascular disease and heart attacks. The real culprits are dental plaque and oral bacteria, which enter the bloodstream and trigger the liver to produce a heat-damaging (inflammatory) enzyme called C-reactive protein (CRP). Cavities and periodontal disease predispose individuals to low-grade chronic infection, which can infect the heart.

Tooth-decay lesions (pre-cavity) are holes in the enamel caused by acid leaching of calcium from enamel crystals. This loss of calcium is somewhat mitigated by saliva, which is calcium-rich and can actually replace small amounts of calcium in enamel crystals. Gingivitis (inflamed gums) results from long-term effects of plaque deposits, which cause irritation and inflammation, rendering gums swollen and tender. This can also be caused by injuries to the mouth, diabetes, pregnancy, illness, heavy metals, and pharmaceutical drugs. Herbal astringents are needed to tone gum tissue. The following mouthwash can relieve gingivitis and retard tooth decay, especially if used just before bed.

Mighty Mouthwash

Fill a one-ounce dropper bottle halfway with:

2 parts tincture of oak bark

1 part each: tincture of myrrh (*Commiphora molmol*), chamomile, sage, and neem leaf

Fill the rest of the bottle with distilled water.

Add 3 drops of each pure, high-quality essential oil: tea tree oil, cinnamon, clove, plus **2 drops** of thyme; and sweet fennel.

Shake well before using; add a dropper-full of mouthwash solution to a small glass of water to use as a gargle, or take straight in the mouth and swish to cover gums and teeth before spitting it out. Doing this before bed will keep plaque from settling in at night.

Skin

Skin or epidermis is our body's largest organ, with more capillary surface than the heart or lungs. Like the earth's surface, whether places are crusty or soft, our skin is responsible for protection and cleansing. It secretes anti-microbial substances, while harboring a friendly community of resident bacteria, which protect our skin from invasion by unfriendly microorganisms. Avoid antibiotics, antiperspirants, and chemical skin products, which can disrupt the delicate balance of these bacteria. In close relationship with the lungs and kidneys, our skin (sometimes called the "third kidney") is actively engaged in discharging impurities from the body all the time. Like the lungs, skin absorbs oxygen and expels carbon dioxide, and, like the kidneys, it excretes organic wastes and salts.

You have approximately seventeen square feet of skin surface! The entire surface is impregnated with millions of sweat glands, which constitute a vast drainage system whereby the blood purifies itself of poisonous waste that it has collected from all cells. When your skin's capillaries are fully dilated, it has six times the capillary surface area of your lungs. This capillary network is required for nutrition and oxygenation of skin tissue, regulation of body heat, distillation of waste from the blood, and exchange of oxygen and carbon dioxide between blood and atmosphere, and is crucial to the heart for normal circulation.

Stimulation of the lymph system greatly aids our skin and vice versa, since any blockage at the superficial lymphatic level will result in congestion throughout the whole lymph system. Skin brushing is an excellent way to address the health of both skin and underlying lymph vessels. Skin also contains millions of nerve endings, which greatly influence overall nervous system activity. This is why skin brushing, receiving a massage or gentle touch can decrease muscular tension, improve lung capacity, digestion, bowel movements, circulation, lymph drainage and promote clear thinking! The top layer of skin, or epidermis, is thin, at only ⅛ inch (3mm). What makes skin "tough" or "thicker" is the dermis, a collagen matrix supporting it underneath, plus the layer of fat below that.

When dermis ages, its connective tissue fibers become rigid, lose resilience and even break into pieces. This causes the support muscles of the skin to lose tone and volume, resulting in dehydration, collapsing and sagging of the skin creating wrinkles and lines. Water, proper nutrients and stimulation of the skin help increase and regenerate production of collagen and elastin fiber. The oil secreted by the sebaceous glands coats the surface of the skin and prevents excessive water loss. Sweat gland function often decreases with aging and strong soaps continually strip the skin of precious oils and acids. Cellulite occurs where fibrous nodules surround fat cells, giving skin a typical orange peel appearance. Cellulite formation is related in part to local vein and lymph congestion.

New skin is grown every twenty-four hours and is as clean as the blood underneath it. Treatment of the skin always requires treatment of other elimination organs because the skin is the last organ in the chain of elimination. Some skin types are more prone to problems than others, but in general, skin reflects the state of our internal chemistry. Blood cleansing herbs categorized as alteratives, such as burdock root and seed, dandelion root, yellow dock, bloodroot serve to clear and strengthen the skin, as do many of those listed under lymphatic care (see chapter nine). Rose hip oil, avocado oil (and pulp), jojoba oil, violet flower oil, essential oil of immortal (*Heliochrysum*) and vitamin E oil reduce scarring in skin recovery.

The skin is cleansed by cleansing all body systems, thus purifying the blood. Renew skin by doing a bowel cleanse, a liver cleanse, and then a kidney cleanse and follow up with a whole food, vegan diet that comprises two raw foods meals and one cooked meal a day. While on the vegan diet, do ten days of the basic liver-flush with a liver decoction each morning followed by a skin-cleansing tea taken throughout the rest of the day (liver tinctures with milk thistle, burdock, dandelion and sarsaparilla can also be taken), take four days off of the flush drink and teas while staying with the vegan diet, then resume ten more days of flushing, and repeat this one more time if you wish. All the while, continue skin brushing, cleansing baths, saunas, bodywork and deep breathing and vigorous exercise.

Skin-cleansing Tea

Equal parts of nettle, red clover (*Trifolium pratense*), mullein leaf and flower, dandelion leaf, calendula flower, hyssop (*Hyssopus officinalis*), horsetail, blue violet (*Viola odorata*), cleavers, and peppermint.

Prepare as a long infusion by steeping, covered, 6 – 12 hours. Drink 3 cups a day.

You'll notice toxins eliminating from the skin, sometimes showing up as pimples, rashes, or boils. This is a sign to keep going until toxins clear out. Application of clay-seaweed masks and body wraps will speed the process. A flaxseed and yarrow poultice and herbs taken internally, such as wild indigo (*Baptista tinctoria*), mullein, lomatium root, red sage root / dan shen (*Salvia miltiorhiza*), and pasque flower will help push out boils. Soon your skin will feel renewed and revitalized!

Help for Common Ailments

Anemia

Anemia or iron deficiency does not always show up on blood tests, since our liver stores iron and it is only when these stores are nearly depleted that blood tests may show abnormally low hemoglobin levels. Symptoms of "depleted blood" include pale skin, nails that are rigid and brittle, wiry hair, constant fatigue, sore tongue, cracks in the corner of the mouth, dark rings under the eyes, pale / chalky stools, weak appetite, and weak immune system. The same foods and beverages discussed above — those that pull minerals out of our bones — inhibit the uptake of iron as well. The treatment of anemia requires foods that are rich in vitamin C and iron, such as citrus, strawberries, cherries, black currants, apricots, raisins / grapes, mission figs, bananas, blackstrap molasses, carrots, almonds, walnuts, leafy greens (especially parsley and spinach), beet root and leaf, sprouts, algae and other super-foods, watercress, artichoke, kelp, legumes (especially red kidney beans), and most blood-colored fruits and vegetables.

In nature, iron is paired with either citric acids or high proteins, such as animal flesh, because iron requires very strong stomach acid in order to be broken down and assimilated. Iron in combination with the high calcium levels often found in supplements is not well absorbed. Our body absorbs only 30 to 50 percent of the iron found in most supplements, necessitating large doses, which disturb sensitive stomachs, cause constipation, and can lead to zinc deficiency. If you feel you must take supplemental iron for a short period, as in the case of anemia or pregnancy, which requires about 130mg / day, then chose a liquid form (Floradix brand is best) and take it before meals with a squirt of yellow-dock tincture in a glass of juice, preferably orange, pineapple, or grapefruit. Below is a recipe for an iron tonic you can make at home.

Liquid Iron Tonic

Combine **one part** organic blackstrap molasses with **one part** organic raw apple cider vinegar and set aside at room temperature in a dark jar for a day.

Pour **one part** of vegetable glycerin in a saucepan and heat on the stove on low.

Add **¼ part** powdered or finely chopped yellow dock root (or ½ part fresh root), and simmer for 30 minutes.

Remove from heat and strain out root parts (if using a fine powder, do not strain). Once the glycerate has cooled, add it to the cider vinegar/molasses, mix well, and let stand at room temperature for two days, then store in the refrigerator. Take one tablespoon of the mixture once or twice a day before meals.

If you are a post-menopausal woman or a man over the age of sixty, avoid supplemental iron tablets or multivitamins with iron, since elemental iron, which can be toxic, is more likely to accumulate in your tissues. Include natural iron in your diet by ingesting herbs and foods rich in iron, or aid in its absorption, such as yellow dock root, nettle, parsley, mullein flower, chickweed, and alfalfa. Three or more cups of iron-rich tea a day along with two cups a day of carrot, parsley and beet juice (drink one cup mixed with half a cup of water two to three times a day), and a daily intake of super-foods (grasses, spirulina, algae) can turn around an iron deficiency in less than a week.

Iron-rich Infusion

Combine **equal parts** of nettle leaf, alfalfa, chickweed (*Stellaria media*), mullein flower, and hibiscus flower.

Use ¼ herb mixture to 1 part water, and steep for 2 hours or longer (overnight for the strongest infusion).
Drink 3 to 6 cups a day, adding 20 drops of yellow dock tincture per cup, for 6 days; then skip a day and repeat.

Plant "blood," chlorophyll, has exactly the same molecular structure as animal blood, except magnesium is its central molecule instead of iron. Thus chlorophyll is the very best blood builder in nature. Greens such as wheat grass, oat grass, barley grass, spirulina, kamut, blue-green algae, alfalfa, cilantro, parsley, dandelion, and spinach, etc., are all very iron-rich. Caffeine, especially that found in black tea and coffee, inhibits iron absorption and should be avoided completely. As always, looking at causative factors is key. Remember that menstruating women lose an average of 15 – 30 milligrams of iron per month and must ingest iron-rich foods and more water to rebuild blood. The ingestion of animal flesh, especially red meats of deer, lamb, and cattle, can also build our blood. If you choose to eat meat, be sure it's organically raised, and keep portions small for easier assimilation. People with low copper levels or low thyroid function (hypothyroidism) often have low iron levels as well. Some people have a low production of certain blood proteins that serve to bind iron, so extra B vitamins (especially B_{12}) may be required. "Getting enough," whether food, rest, or joy, and "feeling enough," also play a role.

Arteriolosclerosis

Arteriolosclerosis is a thickening and hardening of the artery walls from the accumulation of fats and deposits of plaque and cholesterol on the inside of them. This leads to a restriction of blood flow to all cells of the body, especially the heart and brain. When this happens to vessels in the eye, cataracts and macular degeneration result. Arteriosclerosis is primarily a result of lifestyle choices, and is one of the most common causes of death in industrialized society. This condition is treated first by eliminating plaque-forming foods from the diet, essentially those high in cholesterol and those that thicken the blood, such as saturated fats, cooked oils, and animal products — especially fatty meats, high-sugar foods, and cheese. Regular use of herbs such as garlic, cayenne, hawthorn berries, yarrow, red clover, and lime blossom help reduce the accumulation of fat deposits. Daily aerobic exercise is very important, as is cleansing the bowel and liver to remove excess mucus and cholesterol stored in your liver and intestinal lining. Arteriolosclerosis results in a rigidity of internal tissues, which sometimes accompanies an attitude of stubbornness and a "hardening of the heart." Therefore, consider whether you may be currently holding an attitude that is inflexible to change, and whether you are unable to forgive someone. Opening up to reconciliation can help address this condition.

Arthritis

Arthritis is an inflammatory response by the body to a buildup of toxins or mineral salts that have accumulated in joints. The acidity of blood figures into any illness, but particularly with arthritis, since acidic blood keeps the body from repairing. Eliminate from your diet acid-forming foods such as red meat, milk, cheese, alcohol, coffee, black tea, chocolate, aspirin, baked goodies, and sugar — *and don't smoke.* Adopt an alkaline diet rich in vegetables and vegetable protein, and drink plenty of filtered or distilled water throughout the day. Very often, arthritis is an allergic reaction to plants of the nightshade family, which includes potatoes, pepper, chilies, tomatoes, and eggplant. Eliminate all forms of these foods for three weeks and see if symptoms improve.

A quick way to alkalize your blood is to practice deep breathing, exercise joints regularly, drink plenty of water with a squeeze of lemon juice (sprinkle lemon on all grains and proteins before eating), and take regular doses of apple cider vinegar. Vegetable juices, kudzu root mixed with water, and umeboshi plum paste also alkalize blood.

Two of the primary herbs for treating arthritis are burdock root, which moves toxins and excess acids out of the blood, and turmeric, which cools the liver and is anti-inflammatory. Both are seasonally available as produce for adding to soups or making a fresh root tincture. Blood cleansing (bowel, liver, kidneys) will work wonders at relieving not only symptoms, but much of the cause. Some of the strongest anti-inflammatory (thus pain-relieving herbs) are white willow bark, devil's claw tuber (*Harpogophytum procumbens*), evening primrose oil, galangal (*Alpinia officinarum*), ginger, turmeric, Baikal skullcap, rosemary, feverfew, holy basil, and green tea. Digestive enzymes high in protease, including bromelain and papain, taken between meals and at night, can also reduce inflammation. Hormone balance can also play a big role in bone and joint deterioration and inflammation (see chapter seven).

Daily exercise, water therapy, laughter, connecting with nature (especially sunshine), and meditation all help relieve symptoms.

Herbs especially beneficial for arthritic conditions are celery juice, devils claw tuber, prickly ash bark (*Zanthoxylum americanum*), black cohosh, eleuthero, American ginseng, marshmallow root, plantain, rehmannia root (*Rehmannia glutinosa*), burdock root, dandelion root, meadowsweet, yucca root (*Yucca shidigera*), horsetail, white willow bark, boneset herb, boswellia (*Boswellia carterii* or Indian frankincense), ginger, licorice, European angelica, and Chinese angelica (*Angelica sinensis*). Good essential oils for external use are cinnamon, ginger, clove, birch, bergamot, cedar, juniper, frankincense, myrrh, petigrain, and rosemary.

Blood 'n Bones Decoction

2 parts each: white willow bark, devil's claw, and burdock root

1 part each: prickly ash bark (and / or ginger), eleuthero, sliced turmeric, licorice, and juniper berry

Prepare as a decoction or make a tincture.
Drink three cups a day, or take 40 drops of tincture in warm water four times a day.

Bone Spurs

Bone spurs are deposits of excess calcium along the spine or a joint where the body feels it needs more stabilization. They usually occur in areas where there is skeletal stress due to repetitive motion or overuse of a joint. They can reduce and completely dissolve once stress to the area is alleviated and tissues are cleansed. Blood cleansing, bodywork, and teas or poultices that contain "dissolving herbs" such as figwort (spp.), burdock root, gravel root (*Eupatorium purpureum*), cleavers, hydrangea (*Hydrangea aboracens*), uva ursi, sea vegetables, purslane (*Portulaca oleracea*), parsley root, celery root, and turmeric all work to this end.

Eczema and Rashes

Eczema and rashes benefit from a very *simple* whole-foods diet, especially where food allergies are involved. Common food allergens are dairy, wheat, corn, sugar, and citrus. Skin outbreaks are often a sign of unexpressed stress, worry, anger, or sensitivity to one's environment. Rashes are more often a response to heat (internal or external), or to topical exposure to chemical irritants — including poison oak or ivy.

Herbs that relieve itching are chickweed, plantain leaf, grindelia / gum weed (*Grindelia* spp.), calendula, usnea lichen (*Usnea* spp.), club moss (*Lycopodium* sp.), tea tree oil, walnut bark, manzanita bark, propolis, apple cider vinegar, and oak bark. Any of these remedies can be applied topically as a spray-on tincture or salve, or used in a tepid baking-soda bath, while also taken internally. Mix clay and water with one or more of the above herbs to form a thin paste that can be applied to relieve inflammation and itching. A clay poultice will also draw out toxins and oils and keep an insect or spider bite, or poison oak or ivy reaction from spreading.

For cradle cap or other rashes, try soaking the area, using a warm poultice or a bath with a strong measure of the following:

Cradle Cap

---

2 parts chickweed herb (fresh is best)
1 part each: calendula flowers and plantain leaf

Steep, covered, for 20 minutes.

Topical application of rescue remedy can serve to address underlying emotional issues. Taking these blood-cleansing herbs internally will help most skin conditions: burdock root, nettle, cleavers, echinacea, red-clover flower, figwort, yellow dock, Oregon grape, licorice, aloe, chamomile, chaparral, red root (*Ceanothus* spp.), horsetail, milk thistle, rosehip, wormwood, sassafras

(*Sassafras albidum*), sarsaparilla, and dandelion. Be sure to eat plenty of red and dark fruits, vegetables, and herbs, and *drink plenty of distilled or filtered pure spring water*!

Gout

Gout is caused by a concentration of uric-acid crystals in joints (especially fingers and toes), which causes pain that feels "like glass shards." This is a sign of more uric acid in the blood than the kidneys can properly eliminate. There is often a hereditary propensity to gout, but alcohol consumption (particularly beer) is a common culprit. Improper digestion of protein plays a role, so high-protein foods and foods high in purines (which the body metabolizes into uric acid) are often triggers. Therefore, avoid foods such as anchovies, caviar, sardines, shellfish, asparagus, cauliflower, dried beans, herring, meat, oats, mushrooms, and mussels. In addition, stop all consumption of coffee, black tea, alcohol, and very rich foods. Niacin supplements may also precipitate an attack of gout, since nicotinic acid competes with uric acid for secretion from the kidneys.

Many herbs and foods that treat arthritis also treat gout, particularly celery seed, turmeric, boneset, grape seed, pine bark, yarrow, and boswellia. Black cherries and their juice (or concentrate) have been used for centuries to treat gout successfully, as well as blueberries, huckleberries, and strawberries. The enzyme bromelain, found in pineapple, or protein-digesting enzymes containing protease, taken between meals, will reduce inflammation by breaking down excess proteins.

High Cholesterol

Cholesterol, the most abundant steroid in animal tissues, is abundant in our brain, adrenal glands, and nerve-fiber sheaths. It is involved in the formation of hormones and bile salts, and the transport of fats in the bloodstream to tissues throughout the body. Our liver produces cholesterol using essential fatty acids from a wide variety of foods. Some cholesterol is absorbed directly from such cholesterol-rich foods as egg yolks, meat, and dairy products. Egg yolks that are soft (poached, soft-boiled, or fried eggs) contain active lecithin that helps the body break down the cholesterol present, whereas the lecithin in cooked egg yolk is deactivated, leaving our body less able to process cholesterol, thus causing raised cholesterol levels. Cholesterol levels are most affected by diet and stress, or large amounts of caffeine, which mimic stress, but hereditary and metabolic diseases like diabetes are also factors.

Cholesterol is carried in the form of high-density lipoproteins (HDL), low-density lipoproteins (LDL) or very low-density lipoproteins (VLDL). HDLs are protective to the circulatory system whereas LDLs and VLDLs oxidize more readily, thus causing disease. The most effective way to lower cholesterol is to stop ingesting animal products of any kind and replace those fats with omega-3 oils found in nuts and seeds, particularly flax, macadamia nut, coconut, avocado, and soybean. The next step is to flush and clear the liver (after cleansing the bowel, of course!), since that's where excess cholesterol is stored and from which any buildup will continue to be released into the bloodstream. Meanwhile, cholesterol-clearing herbs can be taken.

Cholesterol-clear Tincture

3 parts artichoke thistle

2 parts each: red clover flower, garlic bulb, and dandelion root

1 part each: burdock root, gingko, olive leaf, ginger, and cayenne pepper, plus lemon and / or orange essential oil (or use citrus rind)

Make as a tincture and take three times a day before meals. Do not take this formula if you are on blood-thinning drugs.

Guggul (*Commihora mukul*) is a resin from the myrrh tree used extensively in Ayurvedic medicine for lowering LDL and triglycerides while also raising HDL. It also appears to protect the heart from damage by free radicals. Moving your lymph, whether by skin brushing, hot and cold water therapy, a juice fast, or massage will also help clear cholesterol (see chapter nine).

Hypertension or High Blood Pressure (HPB)

Blood pressure is tension in the arteries maintained by contraction of the heart versus any resistance from the arterioles and capillaries. It is influenced by the elasticity of arterial walls (the less elastic the more resistance, thus the higher the pressure) and thickness of the blood. High blood pressure is treated by taking herbs and foods that increase vessel elasticity while also thinning blood. Herbs and foods that increase vessel elasticity were mentioned earlier, while blood-thinning herbs are listed below under "Strokes." All-important is a consistent exercise program combining strength with flexibility: swimming, martial arts, yoga, dance and aerobics, brisk walking, and stretching, all of which are best when combined with calming the mind — even fifteen minutes a day of centering meditation can lower blood pressure significantly.

Stress has a major influence on blood pressure, because under stress the body deposits more cholesterol on artery walls, and the brain releases chemicals that signal the body to *raise* blood pressure. Lowering the stress in your life by reducing stress factors, or changing your response to them, is as important as taking herbs and foods to lower blood pressure. Remember that substances containing caffeine and high levels of sugar create a stress state in the body by over-stimulating the adrenal glands.

Blood pressure will self-regulate to healthy levels over a period of time when lifestyle changes are consistently applied. One of the "wonder herbs" for regulating blood pressure (either too high or too low) is cayenne pepper. Taken daily in food (building up to more than half a teaspoon two to three times a day) or in capsule form (two capsules two to three times a day) it will lower high blood pressure or raise low blood pressure over months.

Hypertension can also be the result of increased thickness (arteriosclerosis) of the renal arteries, which bring blood into the kidneys to be filtered, or general kidney insufficiency, which causes fluid buildup (edema) in the body (see chapter six). Such fluid imbalance results in excess pressure on the vascular system in general and the heart in particular. The kidneys can be activated by taking mild yet highly effective herbal diuretics such as dandelion root and leaf, nettle leaf, or juniper berry. Essential oils of ylang ylang, lemon balm, and yarrow are calming to the heart and reduce blood pressure.

Low Blood Pressure

Low blood pressure may be hereditary and is usually the result of sluggish circulation, so physical movement is needed — lots of it! A diet that includes plenty of hot and spicy warming foods helps, along with hot and cold therapy to tone your blood vessels. Herbs and foods that distribute circulation include gingko, prickly ash bark, gotu-kola, hawthorn berry, ginger, cayenne pepper, black pepper, yarrow, licorice root, American ginseng (*Panax quinquefolium*), peppermint, apple cider vinegar, and sea vegetables. For poor circulation that leads to chilblains (burst capillaries in fingers and toes), ointments with cayenne, wintergreen, ginger, or mustard, applied to hands and feet, will stimulate circulation. Eating blue, red, and black berries will repair and strengthen capillaries. Occasionally, low blood pressure is caused by hypothyroidism (see chapter six) and should be addressed accordingly. Essential oils of clove, ginger, juniper, cardamom, and black pepper applied topically work well.

Osteoporosis

Osteoporosis, or loss of bone mass, can be alleviated through lifestyle changes and high intake of plant calcium, phosphorus, and magnesium. Plant minerals can be acquired from carrot-beet juice, nettle, horsetail, red raspberry, rosehip, comfrey leaf, oatstraw, sesame seeds, almonds, walnuts, sunflower seeds, soybean, apricots, and leafy greens. One cup of steamed organic kale has as much calcium as one cup of milk — and collard greens have even more! Plant calcium is more readily assimilated and contains the perfect ratio of calcium to phosphorus (2:1), whereas dairy products have a 1:1 ratio, which is not ideal. The dairy calcium in organic kefir and nonfat yogurt is easier to assimilate than the calcium in high-fat diary foods. A diet high in protein, fat, and sugar, along with a sedentary lifestyle, is a primary reason for osteoporosis being so common in industrialized nations. Keep to a diet of mostly plant-based protein, low in saturated fat and devoid of simple sugars. Reduce your intake of foods and drinks that rob the body of calcium, such as coffee, black tea, carbonated beverages, alcohol, salt, sugar, and steroid drugs, and drink this tea:

High-calcium Tea

3 parts each: oatstraw, red raspberry, and alfalfa

2 parts each: nettle, horsetail, comfrey leaf, and spearmint

1 part each: rosehip and damiana leaf (*Turnera diffusa*)

Steep, covered, 30 minutes or longer. For a fully nutritious infusion, soak overnight to drink the next day.

Supplementing calcium is not an unnatural activity; many mammals supplement their diet with chalk, shells, bones, and water high in mineral content — our ancestors did this too! Coral calcium from ancient coral reefs is considered an easily assimilated supplement when dissolved in water, providing the full range of essential trace minerals. A high-quality calcium-magnesium-vitamin-D_3 supplement (your body must convert vitamin D to D_3), bound with herbs or chelated with amino acids, can be of great benefit when needed. Since bone is made of mineral crystals imbedded in collagen (a protein matrix), getting trace minerals such as boron, silica, copper, and zinc (available in sea vegetables), and vitamin D (available in fish, especially sardines, and sunshine on your skin) is necessary for building bone along with easily assimilated proteins. Herbs such as boneset, yarrow, mullein, and comfrey are excellent aids in building bone. Estrogenic herbs and foods (see chapter seven), foods high in vitamins E and C, and those that support the kidneys / adrenals and thyroid / parathyroid are also important for maintaining the skeletal system. Finally, all the care for your bones won't help without regular weight-bearing exercise. Many studies show that bone mass can increase appreciably with regular weight-bearing exercise, even after the age of seventy — it's never too late to start!

Strokes (*Thrombosis*)

Strokes are the result of hemorrhage or blockage of a blood vessel to the brain, leading to lack of oxygen in the brain. Symptoms vary from paralysis of a limb, to loss of speech, to general weakness, depending on which part of the brain is affected. Strokes more often occur where there is thickening of blood, poor circulation, or atherosclerosis, and may result from pharmaceutical drugs. A tendency toward strokes can be mitigated by eating foods high in salicylates, eating plenty of garlic, and using blood-thinning herbs such as red clover, gingko, cayenne pepper, rosemary, beet root and leaf, citrus, vitamin C, and foods high in vitamin E (e.g., avocados, wheat germ, and coconut). *Do not take large doses of blood-thinning herbs if you're on blood-thinning medication*!

A daily glass of fresh-squeezed orange or grapefruit juice thins blood and strengthens blood vessels, as does making sure you get plenty of green food—herbs such as nettle, oat grass, wheatgrass, and alfalfa. As with all circulatory ailments, avoid foods that cause platelet aggregation, particularly sugar and fried, hydrogenated, or baked oils. Recovering from a stroke requires whole foods, vegetable juices, and herbs appropriate to the condition, along with consistent physical therapy. Many people recover fully or at least partially from stroke damage. When a clot occurs in one of the veins of your leg, the condition is called phlebitis, and results in local inflammation. Phlebitis can be treated topically with poultices of arnica flower, comfrey leaf, calendula flower, yarrow, or birch leaves, along with ingestion of herbs and food mentioned above.

Rheumatism

This autoimmune condition causes intense inflammation of the joints; thus treating the immune system (spleen, lymph, thymus, adrenals) is primary (see chapters nine and ten), along with using the anti-inflammatory herbs mentioned above. Any substance depleting to the immune system or agitating to the nerves should be dropped (this includes behavioral and emotional habits as well). Ashwaganda root (*Withania somnifera*) is excellent for nerve and immune-response balance. Flare-ups often occur with emotional upset, hormone imbalance, and other forms of stress. Biofeedback, meditation, yoga, and other means of stress reduction will help.

Adaptogenic herbs such as codonopsis root (*Codonopsis pilosula*) cordyceps fungus (*Cordyceps sinensis*), and other medicinal mushrooms. Fo-ti, Japanese knotweed, Rhodiola (*Rhodiola rosea*), and eleuthero can greatly assist in general support.

Varicose Veins

Varicose veins are a thinning and collapsing of venous walls, which also includes hemorrhoids. This condition typically results from the constant pressure of standing, excess body weight, or carrying extra weight in pregnancy. Venous walls are thinner than those of arteries, and so require toning and strengthening. Alcohol consumption weakens blood vessels, and venous walls in particular. All the foods helpful to the heart are important, particularly those high in *rutin.* Apple cider vinegar is helpful taken internally, but also works well externally in the following combination.

Topical Toner

Combine equal parts apple cider vinegar, tincture of witch hazel (*Hamamelis virginiana*) and tincture of horse chestnut (*Aesculus hippocastanum*) and mix well; add cypress essential oil as desired.

Use cotton balls to apply directly to the skin where you see raised veins.

Herbs such as horse chestnut, collisonia (*Collisonia canadensis*), also referred to as stone root, grape seed extract, butcher's broom (*Ruscus aculeatus*), rosemary, huckleberry, buckwheat, plantain leaf, gotu-kola, horsetail, yarrow, and prickly ash bark can be taken internally as teas or tinctures, in capsules or in food, to strengthen vessel walls and move blood. It's a good idea to elevate your legs for at least one hour a day. Inversion poses in yoga (shoulder stand, headstand, or lying down with your back on the ground and your legs up against a wall or resting on a chair) will greatly assist venous blood flow back to the heart while you relax.

Especially useful is *hot and cold water therapy* (your home tub or shower being "the spa"). Alternating between hot and cold (if your heart is fragile, avoid extreme temperatures) strengthens circulation by causing blood vessels to squeeze and release. Additionally, alternating hot and cold baths, with a bit of mustard powder in the hot bath, does well to stimulate venous flow in the legs. Finding your ideal body weight and maintaining it will also reduce strain on the vascular system. Mix a carrier oil or lotion with essential oil of cypress, rosemary, lemon, orange, or yarrow, and apply it topically to strengthen veins.

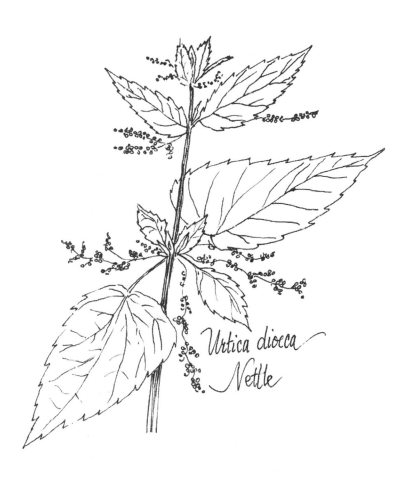

Urtica dioeca
Nettle

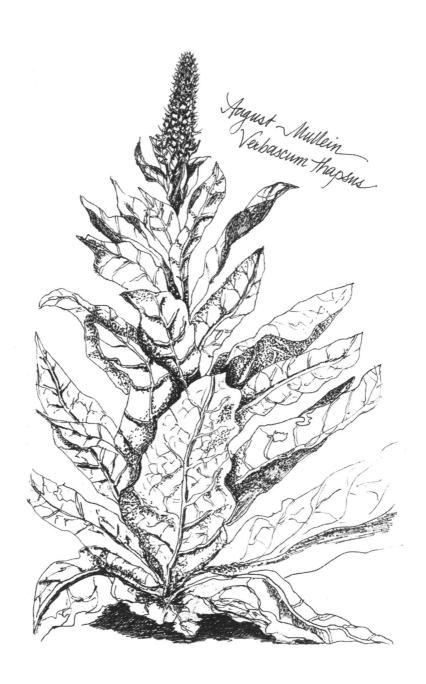

August ~ Mullein
Verbascum thapsus

Chapter Five

The Respiratory System:
Eyes, Ears, Nose, Throat, and Lungs

The essence of becoming a good animal is learning to trust your body.

W. Dyer

The earth is enveloped by a large sac, or ozone layer, which contains atmospheric gases serving as its lungs. Our lungs, and indeed our lives, are directly dependent on the state of the atmospheric conditions that contain us. Air is the great connector with all of life and spirit itself. When we take in the breath of life, we share that air with all life on our planet. Being able to breathe is a gift, from the first breath bringing life into our body, until the last breath we take before leaving. The ocean generates 70 percent of the oxygen we breathe, largely due to enormous amounts of sea vegetation that releases oxygen as a waste product of photosynthesis. Terrestrial foliage provides the other 30 percent of our supply, which is constantly dwindling due to human destruction. Many plant and animal species are currently suffering from this prevailing oxygen debt, and the human species is one of them! We release chemicals into our atmosphere that we wouldn't dream of inhaling, yet we breathe them every day all over the world.

Rosemary
Rosmarinus officinalis

The respiratory and circulatory systems are responsible for supplying our cells with oxygen. This process is controlled by the medulla oblongata in our brainstem — where information is sorted in order to regulate breathing. One-fifth of air is oxygen, which our cells depend on to release stored energy. Oxygen exchange requires vast surface areas: to take up the oxygen we need, our lungs have the surface area of a tennis court! We also breathe through our skin, eyes, and ears. The process of respiration includes breathing air into the lungs, the transfer of oxygen from the air to our blood, the transport of oxygen in our blood to all our cells, the metabolism of glucose inside each cell as it uses the oxygen, and the transport of waste in the form of carbon dioxide to our lungs for expulsion. This process is what provides our cells with the energy they need to live. Respiratory disturbances that inhibit gas exchange in our lungs can lead to low vitality of our body and an increase in metabolic disorders and degeneration of tissue.

Upper Respiratory System

Care of the eyes, nose, ears and sinuses is primarily done by "keeping the windows open and the doors shut." This means breathing through your nose (except during physical exertion and specific breathing exercises), as your nose is the primary filtering system for the lungs. Doing this keeps particulate matter out of the lungs and sinus cavities, as does wearing protective eyewear and ear-wear (earmuffs, hats, and scarves) in windy weather. Mucus functions to trap particles and protect underlying membranes from invasion. Mucus is moved by cells lining our nose and throat, which have little hairs on them (cilia) that pulsate in one direction — toward the esophagus and into the sterilizing acids of the stomach.

These upper respiratory passages, which eventually merge at your esophagus, can be kept clear through the use of pungent herbs like cayenne pepper, horseradish (*Armoracia rusticana*), ginger, onions, and garlic — all the elements of an easy-to-make supertonic! (see appendix for recipe). In addition, the sinuses can be periodically flushed with warm salt water using a netti-pot (a clay vessel used in Ayurvedic medicine, designed to pour salt water through the nasal passages), plus one to five drops of usnea, barberry, Oregon grape, goldenseal tincture, or grapefruit-seed extract if infection is present. Congestion can also be loosened with hot compresses under the eyes and on the brow. For stubborn congestion, there's nothing like herbal snuff!

Herbal Snuff Powder

Equal parts of the following herbs, finely powdered: goldenseal root or Oregon grape root, barberry bark, garlic, and cayenne pepper

Mix well, then put a pinch of the snuff on the back of your hand in the web between your thumb and first finger; hold one nostril closed as you sharply inhale the powder into the open nostril, then repeat on the other side.

The snuff will move up your nasal passage and begin its work, loosening excess mucus and disabling infectious microbes! Do not be alarmed by the stinging sensation — these herbs cannot harm your mucus membranes! With watery eyes, you'll be blowing out loosened material for ten to fifteen minutes. As a general rule, one should only blow the nose when something is ready to come out. Very forceful blowing can push mucus into neighboring sinus cavities, and blowing "up" your nose can spread infection into the upper sinus cavities.

The Throat

The throat is the gateway to our internal organs and thus worthy of protection. It is easily subject to soreness from draining sinuses, straining our voice, food or drink that's too hot, exposure to smoke, stomach acid, inflammation, and infection. Gargling is an excellent way to protect and heal the throat. The following herbs make useful gargles, either as teas or as tinctures added to warm water: sage, oak bark, peppermint, slippery elm, blue violet, thuja (*Thuja occidentalis*), red raspberry, thyme, lemon, goldenseal leaf, arnica, and sea salt. Gargling with echinacea, clove, or kava will provide temporary pain relief by numbing mucus membranes.

Herbs taken as teas or syrups to aid a strained or inflamed throat: elderberry (berry and flower), honeysuckle (*Lonicera fragrantissima* or *L. japonica*), marshmallow root (common mallow root works too), slippery elm bark, licorice, collisonia (good for laryngitis), loquat (*Eriobotrya japonica*), raw honey or honeycomb, propolis or balm of Gilead, comfrey, aloe, and other *demulcents*.

 Herbs that aid an inflamed and infected throat or tonsils: echinacea, garlic, cayenne, agrimony, cleavers, lobelia, myrrh, thyme, tea tree, eucalyptus, elecampane, yerba santa (*Eriodictyon californicum*), lomatium, pine needle, plantain, red raspberry, sage, and thuja. Treating the lymph system will help reduce swelling, especially with the following formula:

 ## Lymph Tonic

3 parts mullein leaf

1 part lobelia

Prepare as a tea, tincture, or compress applied to swollen glands.
Take in small amounts (½ cupful tea or 20 drops tincture) throughout the day, as needed.

It is important to keep your throat covered as much as possible, using a turtleneck or scarf, while it is healing. To relieve a hot, swollen throat, it's helpful to wrap it with a towel that has been soaked in cool mullein tea and wrung out. After it is placed around the neck, wrap it with plastic, then again with a wool scarf or warm towel — this will draw out excess heat and swelling. Remember, however, that swelling indicates a positive active immune response, so do this only in addition to using *diaphoretic* herbs that increase circulation and internal heat: ginger, yarrow, elderflower, or peppermint, for example.

Cough syrups are very soothing, and making your own is easy and fun! You can extract fresh plants such as loquat, honeysuckle, citrus rinds, jasmine (*Jasmine officinale*), rosehip, St. John's wort flower, comfrey, ginger, and elderberry and its flowers, by simply putting the freshly cleaned herbs in a dark jar (or a jar in a paper sack) and covering them with pure vegetable glycerin. Place the jar in a warm place and let the mix soak for at least two weeks — four weeks is even better, and you can keep adding fresh herbs over time. Strain the liquid, then boost its effectiveness with a few drops of essential oils such as orange, tangerine, oregano, or cinnamon. Store in the refrigerator for up to one year. Alternatively, a syrup can be made by simmering herbs in water for twenty minutes, straining, adding more herbs, and repeating this up to four times until the original amount of water is reduced by half. Then add the concentrated extract to the same amount of honey or half honey and half vegetable glycerin. Always be sure to store syrups in a cool, dark place.

The Lungs

Your lungs are the wings of your heart, and in order for them to fly you have to keep them elastic and free from mucus buildup. Deep breathing, aerobic exercise, swimming, singing, and stretching all contribute to long-lasting lungs (and a happy heart). When there is infection or irritation, your body produces more mucus as it attempts to rid itself of cellular waste.

Color and location of mucus is an important factor in determining which herbs to use for moving it. *If the mucus is yellow, brown, or yellow-green, then it is necessary to cleanse the body* by using plenty of lemon, lime, dandelion leaf, turmeric, raw foods and juices, garlic, raw onion, leeks, and diaphoretic herbs that promote perspiration. Drink plenty of body-temperature water. Hot and cold showers, chest rubs (using essential oils of grapefruit, juniper, thyme, eucalyptus), skin brushing, and massage are also important. *If the mucus is white or transparent, then the body needs more heat and energy.* Consume cooked foods, especially hot soups, with warming spices such as horseradish, cayenne, ginger, black pepper, onions, garlic, cloves, and cinnamon. Don't forget hot baths and massage with essential oils of marjoram, rosemary, ginger, and black pepper.

It's important to notice where in your lungs mucus is pooling (upper, middle, or lower). Fluid that is lower in the lungs (if, for instance, one is coughing from the bottom of the lungs) is potentially more dangerous because it can get trapped and provide a perfect environment for growing bacteria and viruses. In natural healing, we want to clear out waste held in mucus by using expectorants, which encourage the loosening and expulsion of mucus up and out of the body. There are stimulating expectorants, which trigger sensory endings in the lining of the bronchioles to stimulate expulsion of mucus. Herbs such as lobelia, white horehound (*Marubium vulgare*), elecampane, propolis / balm of Gilead, yerba santa, osha root (*Lingusticum porteri*), ginger, thuja, and nasturtium leaf (*Tropaedum majus*) fall into this category. There are also relaxing expectorants — these are often demulcents, and serve to loosen mucus by producing thinner secretions, and include herbs such as coltsfoot (*Tussilago farafara*), licorice, slippery elm, comfrey, cherry bark, marshmallow, hyssop, lungwort (*Lobaria pulmonaria*), sundew (*Drosera rotundifolia*), and plantain. Stimulating expectorants are excellent for wet, thick coughs, while relaxing expectorants are good for dry, spastic coughs. Sometimes an apparently dry cough is harboring mucus deep in the lungs, in which case it is helpful to combine both types of expectorants. The above herbs are all toning to the respiratory system in general.

 # Decongesting Decoction

1 part each: osha root, astragalus root, oak bark, cramp bark, slippery elm bark, cherry bark, and ginger

½ part each: star anise, cinnamon bark, black peppercorn, and citrus peel

After simmering for 20 – 30 minutes, strain, add one drop of essential oil of bergamot to every two cups of the decoction. If you like it sweet, add ½ part licorice root or a bit of raw honey.

Building Lung Strength

Weak lungs need lots of calcium, which can be found in the following infusion:

Strong Lungs Tea

1 part each: nettle, red raspberry, comfrey leaf, and plantain leaf

½ part each: licorice, rosemary, horsetail, and yarrow

Any other herbs such as elecampane, yerba santa, lomatium, usnea, pleurisy root (*Asclepias tuberosa*) or elderberry can be added if infection or the threat of infection is present.

Prepare as a long infusion by soaking herbs 2–8 hours.

Plant calcium builds lung tissue and relaxes and strengthens the lungs. It can be found in foods such as barley, carrot juice, dark leafy vegetables, algae, sea vegetables, corn, and cabbage juice. Turnips, also high in calcium, are renowned for their help with lung problems — one remedy calls for making a syrup by cooking turnips in honey.

If you have suffered bronchitis or pneumonia, do not assume it must recur! It just takes commitment and follow-through to strengthen the respiratory system, and to cleanse related systems such as the bowel (a partner of the lungs), and keep the lungs and lymph moving freely. The practice of pranayama (yogic breath), deep breathing of any kind (in clean, fresh air, of course), singing, swimming, chi gong, and yoga all work toward this end. A good formula for strengthening and protecting your lungs is the following:

Lung-tonic Tincture

1 part each: astragalus root, usnea, yerba santa, oak bark, mullein leaf, and blue vervain

½ part comfrey or plantain leaf

The flower essence of comfrey can also be added.

Take 20 – 40 drops in water up to four times per day.

Because lungs pull outside air and particulate matter deep into the body, they are vulnerable to influences likely to upset the balance of the entire body. If defenses are weak, the body's immune response will be unable to effectively ward off offensive pathogens. Symptoms can appear as long-term low-grade fever, chills, and unresolved malaise. This condition is referred to as *wind cold,* which, if it persists over time, can result in chronic illness and exhaustion. If defenses are strong, however, then the strength of the fever will accurately reflect the nature of the pathogen.

If, for example, the pathogen is particularly virulent, then fever will be sudden and high, referred to as *wind heat;* then the body's response will be sufficient to overcome it. In either case, it is your body's own immediate vital response (amount of energy) and immunity that determines the outcome — not just the pathogen itself! A fever assists the struggle against microorganisms, while the act of sweating keeps the temperature under control and speeds up the removal and elimination of toxic debris that would otherwise impact the immune system. The onset of respiratory illness is the time to use diaphoretic herbs to support the body's defense system.

Diaphoretic herbs, also called febrifuges, are active, penetrating and dispersing by nature, and have a dry, spicy, warm taste. While they all promote sweating, some dispel the wind cold condition, and are referred to as *warming,* while others dispel the wind heat condition, and are referred to as *cooling.* Those used to dispel wind cold are helpful when there are infectious internal conditions with acute onset (sensations of chilliness, little or no sweating / fever, muscle aches and pains, and stiff neck). This is the typical condition occurring at the very start of upper respiratory infections. The intention of treatment in this case is to stimulate adequate fever and sweating (increase immune response), so pungent, warming, circulation-stimulating herbs such as cinnamon, ginger, osha root, and yarrow are used. These tend to disperse energy upward and outward like a fountain pushing fluids toward the exterior and out. Of course, all exits (bowel, skin, lungs, and kidneys) must be actively moving wastes out.

Diaphoretic herbs used to dispel wind heat are used when there are few chills, if any, a stronger fever and sweating, and severe inflammation of eyes, nose, throat, and head. In this case the intent is to control and resolve the warmth response before temperature becomes excessive (over 105°F or 45°C), by causing free perspiration (cooling the exterior) and rapid elimination of toxins. Herbs of choice are pungent, cool, vasodilators like boneset, linden flower, catnip, eucalyptus, chamomile, chrysanthemum (*Chrysanthemum x morifolium*), and elderflower. If the temperature remains too high for too long (over four hours in a small child, eight hours in adults), bitter-cool antipyretics (literally "anti-fire" herbs) such as gentian, feverfew, blood root (*Sanguinaria canadensis*), quinine (*Rawolfia caffra*), and quassia bark are useful, as are fresh bitter greens such as watercress (*Nasturtium officinale*), sorrel (*Rumex acetosa*), and dandelion leaves.

If fever is accompanied by aching bones, use willow bark, boneset, or catnip. If fever brings on muscle cramps, there is an imbalance of mineral salts as the body uses them up. Restore salts with potassium broth (see appendix), high-calcium tea (see chapter four), sea vegetables, electrolyte drinks, or Dr. Schussler's homeopathic bio-tissue salts.

Additionally, wrapping the lower legs and feet with ice-cold wet cloths or soaking the feet in ice water will pull fever out of the head, where it is most dangerous. Herbs such as garlic, onion, horseradish, and cayenne can be used in both wind cold and wind heat situations. (To further explore the concepts presented here, see references.)

When our respiratory system is subjected to poor air quality, we must support it with both preventative and post-exposure care. Using throat sprays and taking tonic lung herbs are excellent for this, as is cleansing and building the mucus membranes, while making any appropriate lifestyle changes. If you live or travel where airborne particulate matter is prevalent, you can clear your lungs by making following tea:

Lung-clearing Tea

3 parts mullein leaf

1 part each: peppermint and lobelia

½ part licorice root

Drink three cups a day with 20 – 40 drops of horehound tincture per cup; you can also use two parts horehound leaf in the tea, but using the tincture makes a more palatable tea.

Help for Common Ailments

Asthma

Asthma kills thousands of people in the world each year, and the number grows as air quality decreases. Asthma usually points to a compromised immune system, stressed adrenal glands, and a highly sensitized nervous response to an allergen. Therefore it's important to address the immune system in general and the adrenals and nervous system in particular (see chapters seven and eight). Herbs such as astragalus, ashwaganda root, borage leaf and seed oil, licorice, and eleuthero support both the lungs and adrenals. Nervous-system regulators such as oatstraw and skullcap will also help. If your asthma is caused by allergies, consider taking supplements such as NAC, quercetin, SOD, and homeopathic detoxification formulas to support the liver in its effort to detoxify. It's also important to work the lungs to improve their capacity. Asthma is further aggravated by, and sometimes an indication of, a congested bowel — so consider a bowel cleanse. Asthma can be triggered by environmental factors such as allergies to specific pollens, dairy products, processed grains like wheat or corn flour, animal dander, and especially molds, mildews, and fungi. Many of us live with more mold and airborne fungal spores than we realize. Fungi that survive in dry climates are more enduring and aggressive than those of wetter habitats; however, in wet climates, molds have a way of proliferating that can sometimes run us out of the spaces we live in.

Carefully assess the amount of mold you cohabit with and take steps to minimize it. This entails regular airing of your house and closets (even in the winter), using dry heat, maximizing light exposure, and thorough spring and fall cleaning using organic soaps and natural fungicides such as citrus oils, thyme, oregano, grapefruit-seed extract, sage, eucalyptus, rosemary, lavender, bay, and tea tree. Ward off mildew and moths by placing dried bay leaves and sage in cabinets, drawers, and corners of the room that feel damp. Seal all leaks, and make sure flooring under appliances like the refrigerator and washer stay dry. Burn essential oils of thyme, grapefruit, lemon, eucalyptus, or tea tree in a central room (they will spread throughout the house), or use an atomizer for specific areas such as the bathroom, to dissuade fungal growth. Unfortunately, sometimes one may have to make major repairs, structural changes to a home, or move altogether.

Asthma can also be triggered by emotional stress, especially in children. Therefore, it is always necessary to identify underlying physical and emotional disharmony, which so often accompanies asthma. Where do you need more breathing room? What fears or which person in your life is suffocating you? Bodywork (especially in the thoracic region), spinal adjustment, lifestyle changes, color or sound therapy, relaxation techniques, and flower remedies all come into play. If you have chronic lung problems, especially asthma, it's imperative that you *do not consume dairy products* and other mucus-forming foods such as sugar, most flours, pastas, potatoes, and baked bread products! Many people have eliminated allergies simply by thorough cleansing of the body.

Herbs that naturally dilate bronchioles are lobelia, American ephedra (*Ephedra americanus*, also referred to as joint-pine or Brigham Young tea), yerba matte (*Ilex paraguariensis*), Chinese ephedra or Ma huang (*E. chinensis*), coffee bean, and cola nut (*Cola* spp.). Antispasmodics include grindelia, skunk cabbage rhizome, and cherry bark. Lobelia is both a bronchial dilator and antispasmodic that can help reduce dependency on pharmaceutical inhalers. This is a step-by-step process whereby ten to fifteen drops of lobelia tincture is taken on the tongue whenever one feels the desire to use the inhaler. Lobelia works by relaxing bronchiole muscles, allowing airways to open. Lobelia can lower blood pressure, so it's contraindicated for those with very low blood pressure. Always keep the inhaler nearby for support, and certainly use it if needed. Over a period of two to four months the need for an inhaler will decrease markedly.

Eventually, with dietary and lifestyle changes, cleansing, and follow-through to promote success, many people can put their inhalers away altogether. In a similar manner, lobelia can be used to help quit cigarette smoking, by taking a few drops every time a cigarette is desired, along with high dosages (three to six grams) of vitamin C each day. Stimulating expectorants have the capacity to cause vomiting, which in some cases may be necessary to clear out the lungs; lobelia is such an expectorant, so *keep dosages small.*

American ephedra is a milder bronchial dilator than its Chinese cousin and can be used safely when made as an infusion and sipped by the half-cupful throughout the morning and afternoon (not to exceed two cups a day for adults). The healing herb Chinese ephedra (Ma Huang) has been a source of conflict and confusion due to its misuse and consequent harm to those who have taken it in improper dosages or in combination with the excessive circulatory stimulants in weight-loss supplements. More effective for severe asthma due to its higher levels of ephedrine, Ma Huang is best used with other supporting herbs. Use it for asthma attacks in the following formula:

Bronchial Relief Tincture

1 part each: Ma Huang and lobelia

½ part each: cherry bark, coffee bean, and mullein leaf

8 drops of rescue remedy (Bach Five-flower remedy) per one ounce bottle of tincture

Take this as a drop-dose remedy (1 to 15 drops at a time under the tongue) only as needed with severe bronchial constriction. Never take it in combination with other stimulants such as caffeine, sugar, pseudoephedrine drugs, pharmaceutical inhalers, steroids, high blood pressure, or high blood pressure medications. Use this tincture responsibly on an as-needed basis.

In addition, use the following tea to keep lungs open and clear:

Clear and Free Lung Tea

Equal parts: eucalyptus leaf, holy basil / tulsi, clary sage leaf (*Salvia sclarea*), and juniper berry. Add honey as desired.

If asthma attacks tax your heart, as they often do, then add an equal part of motherwort herb to the mix.

Bronchitis

Bronchitis is inflammation of the bronchi, usually due to bacterial or viral infection the tubes that take air to the lungs. Infection can be triggered by sudden changes in climate, cold, damp air, and a stressed or depressed immune system. Bronchitis should be treated seriously and vigorously in order to prevent more deep-seated illness such as pneumonia. Bring up excess mucus by taking one teaspoon of white horehound tincture three times a day. Keep to a largely fluid diet of hearty soups that contain immune-stimulating foods like shiitake mushrooms, astragalus root, burdock root, lotus root (*Nelumbo nucifera*), garlic, ginger, leeks, onions, barley, sea vegetables, miso, aduki beans, mung beans, root vegetables, and leafy greens. Use immune-boosting herbs as teas and or tinctures: bloodroot, lungwort, thyme, indigo root, thuja, and echinacea (see chapter ten), and keep the lymph system moving with moderate exercise, hot baths, skin brushing, and massage. Chest rubs, warm poultices of ginger or mustard, and castor-oil packs placed on the chest all benefit our lungs and are easy to do. Taking a sauna reduces excess moisture and moves toxins out the skin, so is recommended after bouts of respiratory illness. The following decoction will help clear, soothe, and strengthen lungs:

Lift the Lungs Decoction

2 parts each: osha root, echinacea root, astragalus root, licorice root, and cherry bark (lomatium root may be used in addition, or in substitution for osha root)

1 part each: cramp bark, elecampane root, elderberry, and orange peel

Drink by the half-cupful six times a day until infection has passed and mucus is clear.

Herbal steam inhalation can also help. This includes steam baths or facial steams in which herbs are brought to a boil in water and then taken off the heat to gently emit their essential oils in vapor. Sit with your face over the herbal steam, tenting your head with a towel to keep in the steam. Breathe deeply and relax. This allows the active components of herbs to go directly to respiratory tissues and warms the lungs, thereby loosening mucus build-up. Choice herbs include rosemary, juniper, pine, ginger, thyme, marjoram, lemon balm, lemon myrtle (*Backhousia citriodora*) and eucalyptus.

Ear infection

Ear infection is pain and swelling caused by bacterial or viral infection that has moved up from the sinuses, or as a result of exposure to pathogens in wind or water. Fluid in the ears drains by emptying into sinus cavities, so it's imperative to keep the sinuses open and mucus moving out. Herbs such as mullein leaf and flower, lobelia, calendula, cleavers, and usnea all help move stuck fluids. Take them internally, and apply them externally as compresses to the ear.

Comforting Compress

2 parts each: mullein leaf and flower, calendula flower, and St. John's wort flowering tops
1 part each: lobelia and hops flower, with essential oil of lavender

Steep herbs for 10 minutes and prepare as a compress.

Treat ear infection internally with four drops of ear oil containing oils of mullein, garlic, calendula, and St. John's wort (or make your own by soaking dried herbs in olive oil for at least a month). Apply three drops three times daily and always just before sleep. Most commercial ear oils have some combination of these herbs — always make sure that garlic oil is one of them! Grapefruit-seed extract can also be used as ear drops, and so can most anti-microbial tinctures (glycerin tinctures sting less). A drop of essential oil such as oregano or thyme can be added to ear oil *for adults only* to potentize it. Pressure of the ear, and any obstruction caused by excess wax or particulate matter, can be released by candling both ears using two ear candles per ear and administering ear oil when finished. Repeat every week until your ears clear. Ear oil can also be used the night before candling to help loosen material, as can a light rinse of your ear canal with warm water and apple cider vinegar.

Eye Infection

Treat eye infection by bathing your eyes using the following eyewash:

 ## Bright Eyes Formula

3 parts eyebright herb (*Euphrasia officinalis*)

2 parts goldenseal leaf or root

1 part each: red raspberry leaf, plantain leaf, and chamomile flower

½ part each: milk thistle seed and cayenne

The herb rue (*Ruta graveolens*) can replace cayenne pepper for children's formulas or when using this as a compress.

Eyewash formula is best made as a tincture and diluted in purified or boiled water to use in an eyewash cup or a small glass. Use two to four drops of tincture per eyecup and wash both eyes at least twice per day. This formula can be taken internally as well. If your eyes are red, sore, or puffy, relieve them by placing a slice of cucumber over each eye and resting. Alternatively, a comforting compress can be made with equal parts of eyebright and chamomile. Homeopathic eye drops are also very effective in relieving eye strain and inflammation. Yellowing of the sclera (whites of the eyes) is more often an accumulation of bile in the eye, and can be treated by flushing and cleansing your liver, along with regular eye washing.

Cataracts (*arteriosclerosis of the eye*)

Cataracts occur when the lens of the eye becomes more opaque, so that light rays cannot reach the retina, causing loss of vision. Cataracts may be the result of trauma, extreme exposure of eyes to UV radiation, exposure to chemicals, or viral infection, but more often accompany aging eyes. They are primarily caused by fatty / cholesterol deposits in the eye, and often indicate arteriosclerosis elsewhere in the body. Thus cataracts can be treated by cleansing your bowels and liver, while toning your vascular system in general. To prevent or decrease further buildup of fat on the lens, it's necessary to limit animal fats and heavy oils in your diet. In addition, wash your eyes two to six times daily with the above formula, or try using strained lemon juice in distilled water or saline (2 to 4 drops per eyecup).

Cataracts have become more prevalent because pollution from hydrocarbons interacts with ultraviolet (UV) light and results in the same chemical burn that affects our skin. Wearing good sunglasses and consuming plants rich in carotenoids (yellow and orange pigments) and vitamin C will help protect your eyes. If you're exposed to high levels of UV radiation from traveling, prolonged use of binoculars or scopes in bright sun, or snow and water sports, then supplementation with a twenty-milligram lutein capsule each day is highly recommended.

Macular Degeneration

Macular Degeneration of the retina causes loss of fine, detailed vision, although peripheral vision remains. The macula of the retina is a tiny (three to five millimeter) oval area of the sensory retina, and its degeneration is linked to connective-tissue degeneration and oxidation that often accompanies aging. Herbs that foster connective-tissue strength and circulation to the eyes are helpful: cayenne pepper, rosemary, gingko, skullcap, stone root, horse chestnut, gotu-kola, boneset, prickly ash bark, butcher's broom, sea vegetables, bilberry (and other black and blue berries), rosehip, hibiscus, and red raspberry. Bioflavonoids of all kinds (the natural pigments of fruits and vegetables, which are highly antioxidant) nourish the macula, especially lutein and xanthein, abundant in calendula flower and algae. Supplemental zinc, vitamin C, MSM, and antioxidant combinations, along with herbs for cleansing the liver, can help improve this condition.

Sinus Infection

A sinus infection can be treated with herbal snuff, warm compresses, and netti washes. Add a minute amount of tea tree oil, or a few drops of usnea, coptis, or goldenthread (*Coptis* spp. or Huang lin), goldenseal, or colloidal silver to the salt water in your netti pot. Take the following internally:

Sinus-ease Tincture

2 parts each: usnea, echinacea, any one of the following —
goldenseal, Oregon grape, coptis, or bayberry; and mullein
1 part each: horseradish and lobelia

Prepare as a tincture and take as standard dosage.

The effects of this tincture are amplified when taken with a tea made from
any one or a combination of these herbs: cat's claw (*Unicaria* spp.) pau d'arco,
elderflower, sage, mint, yarrow, aspen, larch (*Larix europaea*), willow bark,
cherry bark, pine needle, or prickly ash bark. As always, boosting the immune
system and maintaining a mucus-free diet by avoiding dairy products, flour,
grains high in gluten (wheat, rye, barley, and oats), and sugar is key. Drink
plenty of water and fresh vegetable juices, and keep respiratory passages moving with daily aerobic exercise. It's important to remember that the sinuses
can also be relieved by treating the ear. Using ear oil can help drain the sinuses
and prevent infections from the sinuses to the middle ear. Ear candling will
remove wax plugs and release pressure on the sinuses. Other helpful herbs
include coptis, stillingia root (*Stillingia sylvatica*), ginger, and any herbs for
moving the lymph system (see chapter nine).

Chapter Six

The Urinary System:
Kidneys, Bladder, and Adrenal Glands

To pee or not to pee, that is the question.

The Earth feels like a solid mass under our feet, but actually is a water planet. With 70 percent water to 30 percent substrate, Earth's topography exhibits the same ratio of liquid to solid as our own bodies do. Water is stored in minerals, soils, and plants just as it is stored in every one of our cells. Large bodies of accumulated water in lakes and oceans are similar to the reservoirs of water in our organs and joints. Connecting all bodies of water are rivulets, streams, rivers, bayous, and rain — just   as all waters of our body are connected in interstitial (between cell) spaces with the plasma of our blood, lymphatic fluid, and the "rain" of moisture taken up by our skin Healthy water, whether in our bodies or in Earth's body, can be characterized by its purity, its richness of oxygen and nutrients, and its ability to flow and cycle, thereby renewing and sustaining life. Water is one of the most conductive substances on earth: it conducts vibrations of sound, light, electricity, and energies around it, and places of healing water have always been revered. In terms of our body's waters, the urinary system is what facilitates storage, regulates pressure, balances electrolytes, and purifies this precious liquid.

Parsley
Petroselinum crispum

Parsley seeds

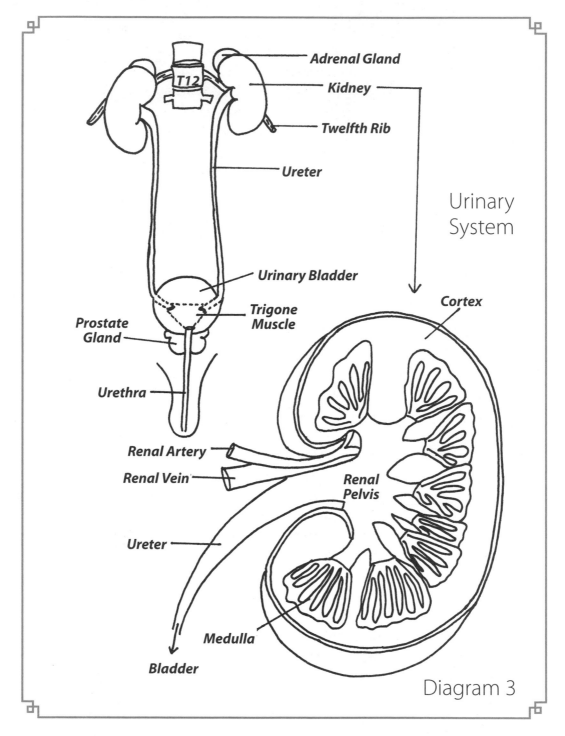

Urinary
System

Adrenal Gland

Kidney

Twelfth Rib

Ureter

Cortex

Urinary Bladder

Trigone
Muscle

Prostate
Gland

Renal
Pelvis

Urethra

Renal Artery

Renal Vein

Ureter

Medulla

Bladder

Diagram 3

The Kidneys

Your urinary system is composed of two kidneys, two ureters, a bladder, and a urethra. The kidneys are indeed shaped like kidney beans (see diagram 3, page 124), and are roughly the size of your fist, weighing about five ounces (141 grams) in an adult. They are located at your mid to lower back (around the 12th thoracic vertebra), nearly covered by the lowest back rib. The right kidney is positioned slightly lower than the left to make room for the liver. In people born with only one kidney, or who lose one, the remaining kidney will double in size as it takes over the function of two.

The renal artery, renal vein, and ureter attach on the spinal side of each kidney. The renal artery brings blood from the body to the kidney to be purified. The renal vein returns the purified blood to the body, while waste in the form of urine (about 95 percent water to 5 percent dissolved substances) exits out the ureter. The ureter from each kidney connects to the bladder, for temporary storage, before elimination from the urethra. Together the kidneys filter an amazing forty-seven gallons (180 liters) of blood each day! This highly efficient filtration system is made up of thousands of nephrons (filtering units) in each kidney, every nephron nested by capillary beds. Useful materials, such as water, glucose, amino acids, vitamins, and minerals, are reabsorbed into your blood depending on how much of those nutrients your body needs. The action going on in the kidneys encompasses much more than filtration. Our kidneys also balance electrolytes, control the pH (acid / base balance) of our blood, and release hormones such as rennin to regulate blood pressure. They also convert vitamin D2 to the active hormonal form of D3, and control the release of aldosterone from adrenals to balance salts.

Ancient healing traditions view the kidneys as storing our body's essential life force; our inherited energy or ancestral chi. They influence the integrity of the bones, particularly knees, teeth, hair, and nails. When we don't replenish our kidneys, their function typically weakens as we age, and therefore care of the kidneys is key to continued vitality. Kidneys are easily stressed by cold, damp weather, too much or too little water, the winter season, fear, anxiety, worry, too little or too much sodium, strong diuretics, prescription drugs (or recreational ones), alcohol, tobacco, carbonated drinks, very particulate or chemically laden water, an overburdened liver or lymph system, constipation, diabetes, and thyroid imbalance.

We eliminate between one and two quarts (up to two liters) of urine a day depending on the amount and types of liquids consumed and how much we exercise (or breathe deeply) and perspire. A noticeable change in the amount of urine eliminated can be a sign that something is out of balance. The look and smell of urine can provide much information about what's going on in our body, and urine has been used as a diagnostic tool for thousands of years. Very dark urine indicates high protein waste, red tones can be a sign of blood, indicating kidney damage (whereas magenta urine is indicative of eating beets!), orange tones point to a bilious or liverish situation, and white strands or milky urine can indicate bacterial infection or excess acid. The odor of urine is also telling. It's a good practice to check your urine periodically so you learn what is "normal" versus unusual for you. By so doing, you'll also learn how various foods and drinks affect your system, and begin to make intelligent choices for your own well-being.

Acidity of urine can be easily checked using pH papers (the multicolor indicators are best) held in urine's mid-stream. While blood has a slightly alkaline pH of 7.35 – 7.45, urine is usually slightly acid with a pH of around 6.8 because the excretion of ammonia captures excess salts and acids. If urine pH is consistently alkaline or severely acidic, it can be indicative of a deep-seated problem. Please note that cleansing and detoxification of the body, or exposure to chemicals, can greatly alter otherwise normal urine pH levels.

Many people take pharmaceutical diuretics for everything from weight loss and edema to high blood pressure; however, nature has provided a plethora of very safe and highly effective diuretics, which, used consistently, along with addressing underlying health issues, will work wonders! The safest diuretics are dandelion root and leaf, leeks, parsley tops and root (*Petroselinum crispum*), carrot tops, nettle leaf, celery seed, stalk, and root, cucumber, watermelon (all melons), fennel, juniper berry, peaches, pineapple, and bilberry / blueberry.

Remember that caffeinous substances like coffee and tea leaves are strongly diuretic and depleting to the body, since they tend to pull out important salts like potassium, magnesium, and calcium, thus upsetting mineral balance. Alcohol is a trick diuretic in that it "fools" the kidneys into activating the hormone aldosterone, which in turn tells nephrons to release sodium. This upsets the balance of tissue salts, resulting in edema, which can eventually raise blood pressure, even though a blood test might show low sodium levels.

For strengthening the kidneys, barley water is excellent and easy to make:

Be Strong Barley Drink

Put ¼ cup whole organic barley in a pot with 2 cups of water (or make any amount using that 1:8 ratio), and a bit of grated ginger and / or cinnamon stick. Cover, simmer for 20 minutes, strain, and add a little lemon or molasses if desired.

Barley water is loaded with calcium and very fortifying to our kidneys and adrenals. Soup made with barley is great too! Other nourishing foods and herbs are whole buckwheat (kasha) or buckwheat sprouts, vitamin B_6 (dark leafy greens / algae, brewer's yeast), shiitake mushrooms, rehmannia root, lycii / gojji berry (*Lycium chinense*), and lotus root.

Foods that strongly activate or cleanse the kidneys are parsley, asparagus, sweet corn, zucchini, carrots, lettuce, cabbage, beets, and dark red / black fruits (all the berries); but avoid asparagus if your kidneys are inflamed or very weak.

Avoid the following if you have a propensity toward kidney-stone formation or have under-functioning kidneys: black tea, coffee, carbonated drinks, chocolate, peanuts, rhubarb, spinach, chard, tomatoes (particularly cooked ones), strawberries, beet root, and red meat. These foods are high in oxalic acid, which irritates tissues and binds up calcium (large amounts can lead to calcium stones). Some of these foods also contain purines (nitrogen-containing compounds that result from the digestion of protein), which are prevalent in meats and dairy, and aggravate the kidneys. Refined sugars and phosphates (especially in sodas) and salt also need to be avoided. Drinking distilled or purified water will reduce stone formation.

Herbs that aid the kidneys can have different actions; therefore, when treating the urinary system holistically, it's helpful to combine herbs of differing actions.

Antiseptic herbs have volatile oils to work on microbes. Some of these are: juniper berry, uva ursi leaf, cranberry (*Vaccinium macrocarpon*), buchu leaf (*Agathosoma betulina*), Oregon grape root, echinacea, plantain, and yarrow.

Demulcent herbs soothe irritable tissues and include: corn silk, couchgrass (*Agropyrum repens*) marshmallow root, and licorice root.

Anti-lithic herbs prevent stone formation or aid in the breakdown of urinary stones. These include herbs like: cleavers, parsley root, carrot tops, goldenrod tops (*Solidago virgauria*), blue flag (*Iris versicolor*), chickweed, gravel root, hydrangea root, lobelia, stone root, butcher's broom, watermelon, and white pond lily (*Nymphaeca odorata*).

Toning herbs include schizandra berry, dandelion root and leaf, pipsissewa (*Chimaphila umbellata*), horsetail, gingko, nettle, astragalus root, and watercress.

A kidney or bladder tea could include a combination of herbs from each category, with citrus peel, peppermint, or ginger added to disperse the herbs and warm the formula. Sometimes microbes infiltrate our urinary system and must be flushed out; the recipes below work well together, and can be taken periodically to prevent infection.

Urinary Clean and Clear Tincture

2 parts each: pre-cooked usnea lichen, uva ursi leaf (manzanita can substituted), parsley root, and marshmallow root

1 part each: Oregon grape root, juniper berry or buchu leaf, and fresh or dried cranberries

½ part lobelia

Make as a half-alcohol, half-vegetable-glycerin tincture that can be added to Kidney-Bladder Tea.

Kidney-Bladder Tea

2 parts each: spearmint, goldenseal leaf, goldenrod tops (carrot tops can substitute), cleavers, corn silk, and horsetail

1 part each: yerba santa, uva ursi, marshmallow, chamomile, and licorice

Prepare as an infusion and steep, covered, for at least 20 minutes. While steeping, add a dropper-full of the above tincture for each cup of tea.

Echinacea tincture or oregano oil can be added to either of the above formulas if your immune system is low or infection has been lingering.

To end urinary-tract infections in four to six days, take 30 to 50 drops of Urinary Clean and Clear Tincture in a cup of Kidney-Bladder tea, six times a day, while following a cleansing (alkalizing) diet that includes probiotics. Always drink *plenty of lemon or lime water* and get enough *rest*. Just before bed, be sure to take unsweetened cranberry juice, or two cranberry capsules, to prevent proliferation of bacteria in the bladder while you sleep. Once you're well, a pleasant tea for maintaining kidney balance is as follows:

Build 'n Balance Kidney Tea

2 parts each: schizandra berry, rehmannia root, and lycii / gojji berry
1 part each: marshmallow, dried cranberry, horsetail, cleavers, and licorice

Let the mix sit overnight in water (one heaping teaspoon of the dry herb mix per cup of water). In the morning, bring to a boil, turn off heat, steep, covered, for 10 minutes, strain, and drink. Add anti-microbial herbs, such as usnea or uva ursi, if necessary.

Whenever we drink purified or excellent spring water in copious amounts (up to one gallon or 3.7 liters per day) we are reducing stone formation and cleansing the kidneys. Periodically drinking distilled water will further reduce stone formation. Good, clean water is what kidneys love most, so make sure that's what you're drinking! Municipal waters are treated with chemicals such as chlorine, bromine, and fluoride, which are damaging to all organs, especially the kidneys. Soft-water systems put the kidneys through a lot of work, and hard water (especially well water) can be high in solutes, causing stress to our kidneys. Even old lead and copper piping can damage these fine organs and cause mineral imbalances in the body. Having your water quality checked and purchasing a water-filter system if necessary is the first step. Most people will greatly benefit by doing a kidney cleanse at least once or twice a year, usually during warm weather, since kidney cleansing tends to cool the body.

 One-week Kidney Cleanse

This cleanse lasts seven days and can be done two to four times a year. If you're treating a bladder infection, start a kidney cleanse immediately! Be sure to have cleansed the bowel within the past two months, but if you need to jump right into cleansing now, then just be sure to take bowel-toning and cleansing herbs and foods to keep wastes moving out of the system. Start each morning with a kidney-flush drink.

Kidney-flush Drink

One pint of purified or distilled water (warm or room temperature) with the juice of one lemon or lime and a dash of cayenne pepper.

Follow this with two cups of Kidney-Bladder Tea with 40 to 60 drops (roughly one teaspoon for an adult) of Urinary Clean and Clear Formula. Drink two more cups of tea with tincture after lunch, and two more cups of tea with tincture after dinner, for a total of six cups of tea and six doses of tincture a day throughout the cleanse.

✻ For two days eat raw fruits, vegetables, soaked nuts, and seeds, with fruit in the morning, vegetables all day and early evening, and fruit at night (separate your consumption of fruits and vegetables by one hour).

✻ Follow with three days of liquids: fresh juices (same sequence — fruit-veggie-fruit) with water. Drink potassium broth and barley water as desired.

✻ End with two days of raw foods, all the while drinking plenty of purified water with a bit of lemon, the tea, and tincture.

✻ When finished, *slowly* introduce steamed vegetables and grains.

✻ It's very important to drink at least a gallon or more of liquid a day!

While cleansing, take time to rest. Be sure to stay warm, get aerobic exercise (*sweat!*), belly-breathe for fifteen minutes each morning and evening, take a sauna or steam bath, and skin brush. Warm (but not too hot) baths with essential oils of cedar, juniper, and lavender are helpful. Warm ginger and juniper compresses, with or without castor oil, can be applied over the kidneys (upper lumbar / lower thoracic spine area) to soothe. Process and record any emotions that arise. A little release of water from the eyes can help your kidneys too — so cry if you feel like it!

Born of water – cleansing – powerful – healing – changing – I AM!

— a nice chant while cleansing

A kidney cleanse can help dissolve and prevent kidney stones, but if you're aware of having stones and want to systematically pass them, do the kidney cleanse and follow up with another two-day liquid fast, drinking the following *Dissolve Tea* each day.

 ## Dissolve Tea

Mix together two cups of the following:

1 part each: hydrangea root, gravel root, and marshmallow root.

In a large container, add these herbs to 3.5 quarts (approx. 3 liters) of fresh-squeezed or bottled organic apple juice (preferably from sour apples), plus 1 cup each: fresh-squeezed lemon and lime juices, and 1 cup raw organic apple cider vinegar.

Let the mixture sit at cool room temperature (50 – 68°F / 10 – 20°C) for 24 hours, shaking it occasionally. You can even mix some or all of this formula in a blender to break it down further. The next day, strain the liquid through a stainless-steel mesh or clean cheesecloth, then sip half a cup (4 ounces) every hour. Alternate this tea with distilled water, drinking as much of both as you can, up to one gallon of each if possible (be sure to finish the tea). This means that you're drinking about a cup of Dissolve Tea and a cup of distilled water every hour throughout the day. Repeat this process for a second day.

The marshmallow root and apple serve to coat any sharp edges of stones, while gravel root and hydrangea root dissolve them. By doing the previous kidney cleanse, stones will be pre-softened and the passageway open for rapid release and efficient elimination. Even so, passing stones and gravel (and they can also come from the bladder as bladder stones) can be very painful. When in the throes of passing stones, take a warm bath with Epsom salts, sea salt, and essential oils of juniper, chamomile, and lavender. As you sit in the tub, sip the following tea, or take it as a tincture in warm water:

Relieve Formula

2 parts each: lemon verbena (*Aloysia triphylla*) and valerian root

1 part each: St. John's wort and blue vervain

½ part lobelia

As you feel the stones passing, allow yourself to eliminate them in the bath.

The Bladder

The bladder can also be subject to stones and infection, and is a common site for cancer. Relieve your bladder when you need to, and know that cleansing the kidneys also cleanses the bladder. Specific problems are addressed below.

Help for Common Ailments

Bladder Stones

Treatment for bladder stones is the same as for kidney stones.

Incontinence

Incontinence can be caused by weakening of the pelvic floor, inflammation of the trigon area of the bladder, obesity, chronic constipation, enlarged prostate, obstructions in the ureter, or stress-related psychological factors. A very helpful combination is the Bladder-toning Tincture below.

Bladder-toning Tincture

6 parts parsley root

3 parts nettle root

2 parts each: black cohosh, blue cohosh, marshmallow root, horsetail, white pond lily, and uva ursi

1 part each: lobelia, rehmannia root, and yarrow

½ part ginger rhizome

Prepare as a tincture, and take for 3 weeks.
Dosages:

> *Children 4 to 8 years — 20 drops twice a day*
> *Children 8 to 12 years — 20 drops three times a day*
> *Children 12 years to adult — one teaspoon three times a day, plus one teaspoon before bed, for a total of four teaspoons (see dosages in appendix for adjustment of this dose to body weight).*

Address any fears, worries, or anxieties: St. John's wort flower remedy can be taken as support for this, or use a drop-dose (energetic dose) of St. John's wort tincture, 2 to 6 drops each morning and just before bed. Other herbs such as comfrey leaf, boneset, and agrimony can help strengthen the bladder's sphincter muscle, as does eating plenty of calcium-rich foods and practicing Kegel exercises (squeezing and releasing the anal sphincter and perineum) and abdominal strengthening exercises everyday. Take relaxing herbal teas (especially in the early evening) with wood betony (*Stachys officinalis*), hops, skullcap, passionflower, kava, wild lettuce (*Lactuca virosa*), and valerian root.

Interstitial Cystitis

Interstitial cystitis is chronic inflammation of the bladder lining. It may be caused by chemical exposure (feminine deodorants, antibacterial soaps), contraceptive creams, diaphragms, holding a full bladder too long, a tipped bladder / uterus (which traps urine), oral contraceptives, leaky gut syndrome, antibiotic use, or stress. With cystitis, it hurts to hold urine in the bladder and it is a relief to pee — *the reverse feeling from a bladder infection*. The mucus barrier on the inner lining of the bladder breaks down, thus the stinging sensation even if a urine pH test shows as alkaline. *Don't flush with acids!* Use demulcent herbs: marshmallow, slippery elm bark, aloe juice, licorice, and corn silk. Grindelia flower, yerba santa, usnea, oregano, and cleavers will help reduce any infection and inflammation. Couchgrass, horsetail, and yarrow will improve cell structure. To stop inflammation, one must consume alkaline foods — all vegetables and very little fruit (avoiding sugar helps), lentils, mung beans, millet, soy, barley, quinoa, amaranth, wheat berries, corn, kelp, algaes, grasses, and raw garlic if you can tolerate it, plus herbs such as thyme, rosemary, basil, and turmeric. Every two hours, drink a cup of the following tea:

River of Relief Tea

Equal parts: dandelion leaf, cleavers, corn silk, yarrow, usnea, skullcap, and finely ground marshmallow root

Steep, covered for 20 minutes and drink up to six cups a day.

Take echinacea for ten days and goldenseal for four days. A warm (not hot) bath with essential oils of cedar, bergamot, juniper, eucalyptus, and lavender helps. If the urethra is inflamed or infected, indicating urethritis, include twice the amount of marshmallow root and topically apply kava kava (put kava tea in a small spray bottle and mist the urethra after each urination). The bladder nerves pass between the 4th and 5th lumbar vertebrae, so spinal adjustments or acupressure can be helpful. Pain can be addressed with skullcap, St. John's wort, marjoram, valerian, blue vervain, and California poppy.

Prostatitis

Prostatitis is an inflammation of the prostate usually caused by infection. Since there is pain upon urination, it can be confused with a bladder infection. You can treat it the same as you would cystitis, but include herbs such as echinacea, saw palmetto berry, hydrangea root, nettle root, horsetail, and angelica. Soaking the penis in a demulcent herb tea made by combining kava with marshmallow or slippery elm bark can provide relief.

The Adrenal Glands

Adrenal glands are endocrine glands found just above each kidney (see diagram 3, page 124). Though our adrenals are not considered part of the urinary system per se, they work with the kidneys in balancing salts (thus fluids), blood pressure, and the release of minerals in the body. Adrenal glands act as "spark plugs" for vitality in our body; they are initiators and regulators, and need to be cared for to ensure our vibrancy late into life. While kidneys store our inherited energy, adrenals help manage how we use that stored energy, and their health is indicative of how we manage our own energies. Each adrenal gland is divided into two regions: the cortex, which secretes hormones that affect metabolism and reproduction, and the medulla, which is part of the sympathetic nervous system and our first line of response against physical and emotional stress.

The cortex secretes several hormones: aldosterone, which inhibits the amount of sodium secreted in urine, maintaining blood volume and pressure, and androgens, which stimulate the development of male sex characteristics and regulate testosterone levels in both sexes. The cortex also secretes hydrocortisone and corticosterone, which control our body's use of fats, proteins, and carbohydrates, as well as suppressing inflammatory reactions. Epinephrine and norepinephrine (both forms of adrenaline) are the hormones secreted by the adrenal medulla in response to stimulation by sympathetic (spinal / brain) nerves, which are most active in times of stress. The release of adrenaline supplies more blood to active muscles by increasing heart rate, which forces heart contraction, raises blood sugar, expands airways, and constricts blood flow to the intestines and organs. This fight-or-flight stress response is meant to release short-term bursts of energy for escaping immediate danger. It is essential that this excess energy be used in physical activity; if adrenaline isn't used, as is often the case with emotional stress or work stress, it circulates internally, causing oxidation of tissues.

Repetitive activation of the adrenals by chronic stress can wear them down and eventually lead to chronic disease. Taking care of our adrenal glands means avoiding substances that initiate a stress response, such as strong stimulants, sugar, drugs, alcohol, and steroids, as well as *reducing and releasing everyday stress*. Even so, environmental and sociopolitical stress affect all of us to some degree, so herbs that nourish and renew our adrenals can be taken three to six days a week. A number of plants, such as borage, ginseng, licorice, maca root, and wild yam, contain the natural precursors (plant steroids) to adrenal hormones. The following formula will help your body adapt to everyday stress with plant sterols that nourish your adrenal glands toward sustainable energy.

Everyday Energy Tonic

2 parts each: wild yam and eleuthero

1 part each: maca root (*Lepidium meyenii*), suma (*Pfaffia paniculata*), licorice root, and gotu-kola

½ part reishi mushroom

Prepare as a tincture or decoction.

Wild yam root, maca root, schizandra berry, eleuthero, cat's claw bark, suma bark, and American, Chinese, or Korean ginseng (*Panax* spp.) are some of the finest tonic herbs for the adrenals. They are adaptogenic, so they help the body adapt to stress while normalizing hormone function. Oils of borage, evening primrose, and black currant are also very restoring to the adrenal glands since their GLAs (gamma linolenic acids) provide building blocks for steroid production. Other adaptogenic, adrenal-restoring herbs and foods include avocados, ashwagonda root, astragalus root, cold-water fish, codonopsis root, jujube date (*Zizyphus jujuba*), wild oat seed, fo-ti or He shou wu, rhodiola, ligustrum fruit, kombu seaweed, Baikal skullcap, and damiana, as well as all medicinal mushrooms such as shiitake, maitake, reishi, cordyceps, and others.

Our adrenal glands store some amounts of vitamins C, D, and E. When constantly stimulated, these stores become depleted. When you're experiencing periods of high stress, give your body large quantities of antioxidants — especially vitamins C, E, and the B family — to help the adrenals. A diet of sprouted, raw foods and juices will give you the greatest vitamin and mineral boost. Antioxidants in grape-seed oil, pine bark, olive leaf, citrus, chlorophyll, supergreens, algaes, all sea vegetables, alfalfa, all the grasses, nettle leaf, milk thistle, organic Brazil nuts (selenium), green tea, and bee products (pollen, propolis, and royal jelly) all feed our adrenals. In addition, try the following decoction:

 ## Adrenal Support Formula

2 parts each: astragalus root, cat's claw, fo-ti (He Shou Wu), reishi mushroom, American ginseng or eleuthero, wild yam, and licorice

1 part each: rehmannia root, schizandra berry, ginger, and orange peel

Make a large, strong decoction by simmering, covered, for 30 – 50 minutes. You can store decoctions up to three days in the refrigerator; otherwise, make as a tincture. This formula can be taken daily.

Restore your adrenals by taking time out to quiet your mind and relax your body. Replenish your energy through meditation, walks in nature, gardening, short naps, play, deep breathing, sex, yoga, daydreaming, chi gong, and any other ways you like to rekindle your inner fire.

Help For Common Ailments

Adrenal Exhaustion

Adrenal exhaustion is a serious condition that comes about when the adrenal glands have been over-stimulated to the point where they're unable to carry out their functions. Early warning signs are inability to sleep, restlessness, poor digestion, allergies, hyperactivity, mood swings, weakness, weight loss, hypo- or hyperglycemia, reproductive problems, more susceptibility to illness, and autoimmune diseases. Note that cumulative exposure to electromagnetic radiation emitted from medical radiation treatments, cell phones, towers, radio towers, and computers can disrupt and deplete function of the adrenal glands. Don't wait until you experience symptoms such as inability to sleep despite constant fatigue. Act now to support your kidneys and adrenals by making necessary lifestyle and dietary changes. Often there's a need to increase protein intake and reduce sugars and simple starches. Cleanse your kidneys as you support the adrenals with the aforementioned herbs and foods, and take time out for rest and relaxation! Remember, it takes a long time for adrenal imbalance to develop, so it requires patience and persistence to restore health and vitality.

Allergies / Hypersensitive Immunity

Allergies and hypersensitive immunity are often signs of overburdened adrenals and liver. Elimination of allergies requires appropriate lifestyle changes, detoxification, herbs and foods for adrenal support, and stress reduction. Stop, or at least seriously limit, exposure to any known allergens. A bowel cleanse containing bentonite clay and apple pectin will help draw out toxins and residual radiation that would otherwise deplete the adrenals over time. Address any hormonal imbalance and consider brain-balancing techniques, cranial-sacral therapy, meditation, yoga, chi gong, and flower or homeopathic remedies. Taking appropriate brain and nervous-system tonics, as teas or tinctures, can help immensely. One of the best herbs for allergies to pollen is nettle leaf taken in substantial quantities (3 to 6 cups of strong tea, or 2 freeze-dried capsules 3 to 4 times a day).

Other herbs and foods for allergy relief are cat's claw, pau d'arco, eyebright, grapefruit seed extract, lecithin, quercetin (the antioxidant pigment found in the peels of red onions, purple garlic, grapefruit peels, apple peel, and eucalyptus leaves). Echinacea can over-stimulate the immune system in those with chronic allergies, but herbs with berberine or hydrastine (Oregon grape, bayberry, barberry, and goldenseal) do well.

Allergies are the body's defensive response to irritation (insect bites, stings, and chemical irritants) or emotional upset, and often show up as skin complaints. Rashes and hives indicate an acute response. Taking lymph-moving herbs such as mullein, blue flag, cleavers, and red root, while also using nervines (herbs that act on the nervous system) such as lobelia, valerian, skullcap, and St. John's wort, will help the reaction pass within three days.

Allergens are usually things we become sensitized to after repeated exposure. Observe your body's response to your environment and what you consume on a daily basis. Allergies develop more frequently to foods we are "addicted" to, those we constantly crave and eat. Daily exposure to molds, dust, and chemicals can cause an allergic reaction over time. For example, excess mucus or lymphatic congestion are common signs of an intolerance for dairy or the gluten protein found in grains. Aching joints, constipation, and inflammation often point to an intolerance to the nightshade family (potatoes, tomatoes, eggplant, and peppers). Environmental allergies from exposure to chemicals of all kinds, petroleum, molds, and radiation, can eventually manifest as a hypersensitive immune response.

Change of habit and habitat reduce the chance of allergy formation because, in nature, variation leads to adaptation. Treatment of allergies involves three parts: boosting the immune system (see chapter ten), strengthening the adrenal glands (herbs mentioned in this chapter and chapter seven), and treatment of specific symptoms (chapter five).

A Checklist for Allergy Treatment and Prevention

Keep the lymph moving — with physical activity, perspiring, saunas, hot baths, skin brushing, salt rubs, hot / cold showers, pungent spices, and lymph-moving herbs.

Keep nasal passages clear — use a netti pot to wash your nose, use herbal snuff, ingest ginger, cayenne, and horseradish.

Keep eyes clear — use eyewashes and herbal compresses.

Keep lungs open — use herbal steam inhalation, herbal bronchodilators, deep breathing, aerobic exercise, and herbs and foods that strengthen and clear the lungs.

Keep the digestive tract strong and the bowels open — use cultured foods, probiotics, bitters, and live foods, and do regular bowel and liver cleansing.

Eat and drink a wide variety of plant foods — especially wild ones! Let food be your medicine and use fresh herbs liberally.

Change your environment — cleanse and clear your living space; travel, alter the way you habitually do things, and periodically review and renew your life.

Dialogue with your inner self — take time to listen to your sacred inner being and body; spend time alone in nature; express yourself through art, writing, music, dance, and pleasurable activities.

Practice positive communication — reprogram your system by noticing what you tell yourself about your health in general and your body in particular. Laugh a lot.

Use energy medicine — never underestimate the power of flower remedies, energy work, homeopathy, and sound and color therapy — and stay open to the unknown!

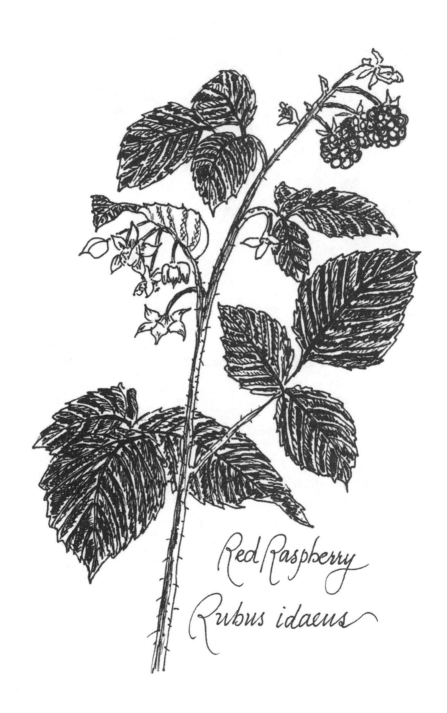

Red Raspberry
Rubus idaeus

Chapter Seven

The Reproduction System:
Endocrine Glands and Hormones

*Exposure to the sun and contact with
the earth brings strength and blessing.*

Native American wisdom

O ur reproductive cycle reflects our connection to natural cycles in the universe. Listening to and honoring our reproductive rhythms brings us closer to the universe inside us. The sun and moon, in particular, affect our hormonal cycles in the same way they affect the earth's tidal rhythms. The movement of stars and the cycling of seasons is an outer picture of the spiral of life unfolding inside us via the rhythms of the endocrine or glandular system. Becoming more aware of celestial cycles awakens awareness to our body's responses to environmental cues, and tunes us into our inherent nature. The reproductive system relies on glands that produce and secrete hormones directly into the bloodstream for nearly instant cellular communication. This feedback system reveals how we feel about ourselves in reference to the world we live in.

Chastetree
Vitex agnus-castus

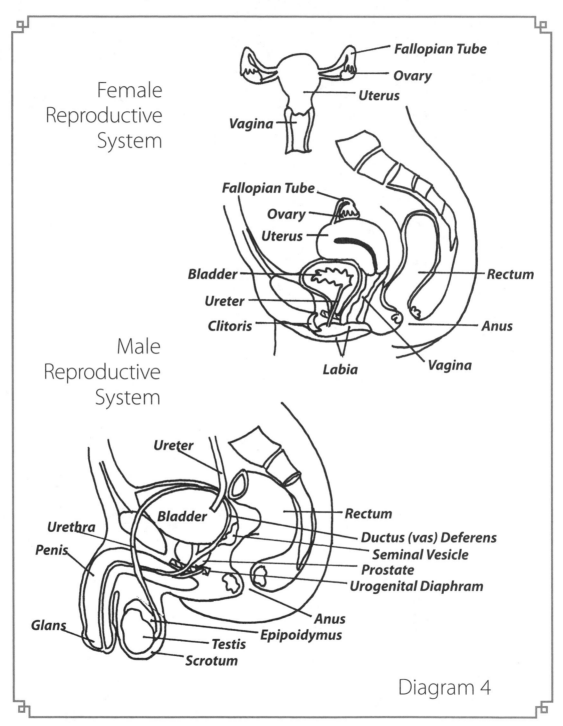

Female Reproductive System

Male Reproductive System

Female Reproductive System labels: Fallopian Tube, Ovary, Uterus, Vagina

Labels: Fallopian Tube, Ovary, Uterus, Bladder, Ureter, Clitoris, Labia, Vagina, Rectum, Anus

Male Reproductive System labels: Ureter, Bladder, Urethra, Penis, Glans, Testis, Scrotum, Rectum, Ductus (vas) Deferens, Seminal Vesicle, Prostate, Urogenital Diaphram, Anus, Epipoidymus

Diagram 4

Nearly all cells in the body have hormone receptors, which serve as a kind of "universal consciousness," coordinating and regulating bodily functions. Here are the primary endocrine (ductless hormone-secreting) glands:

Pineal gland. Located at the top of the brain, this gland produces *melatonin* and is connected with the autonomic nervous system.

Hypothalamus. Located behind the eyes, toward the back of the brain, this is the primary gland regulating hormone release from the pituitary. It produces *oxytocin* (for breast milk production and secretion) and *antidiuretic hormone* (to reduce water loss).

Pituitary. Located just below the hypothalamus, it's the storage and release center for *oxytocin* and *antidiuretic* hormones. It produces *somatotrophins, prolactin,* and *thyroid stimulating hormone* (TSH), along with the reproductive hormones *follicle stimulating hormone* (FSH) and *luteinizing hormone* (LH), plus adrenal hormones (*androgens*).

Thyroid. Located midway along the neck to the front and sides of the trachea, it produces *thyroid hormone* and *calcitonin*.

Parathyroids. This pair of glands attached to either side of the thyroid secrete *parathyroid hormone,* which maintains blood calcium levels by promoting calcium uptake by the kidneys and the release of calcium from bone.

Pancreas. Located behind the sternum, to the back of the body, stretching from duodenum to spleen, this gland secretes pancreatic juice (digestive enzymes), and the hormones *insulin* and *glucagon.*

Adrenals. One is located on top of each kidney; they secrete *androgen stimulating hormone* (AASH), responsible for testosterone and steroid regulation.

Ovaries. Located low in the female pelvic cavity on either side of the uterus, they produce eggs, *estrogens* (estrogen, estradiol, and estrone), *progesterone,* and *testosterone.*

Testes. These two oval-shaped organs that hang below the penis, in a pouch of skin called the scrotum, produce sperm and the hormones *testosterone* and *estrogen.*

Men and women share the hormones estrogen and testosterone, though they're produced and regulated differently. From a physiological standpoint, male and female reproductive systems operate in a similar manner: both are regulated by the hypothalamus and pituitary glands, and rely on the adrenal glands for backup support of hormone production and secretion.

Like other systems of the body, the endocrine system works toward homeostasis (internal balance) by way of individual glands assisting one another. If one gland is impaired, over-functioning, under-functioning, or removed, all others will shift their production and secretion to compensate until balance is restored. Therefore, when treating one gland, it's best to treat the rest simultaneously, in holistic fashion. Glandular function also changes with varying life stages for men and women, and these natural shifts go much more smoothly when supported physically, emotionally, and spiritually.

Both male and female reproductive systems can be cared for in similar ways, using many of the same herbs to nourish and tone. Dysfunction of the reproductive system is largely a dietary and lifestyle problem, in which a lack of exercise and lack of nutrient-rich foods (especially the avoidance of naturally bitter flavors) weakens vital energy. Additionally, environmental contaminants such as estrogen-mimicking xenoestrogens, and phthalates from plastics, have been linked to infertility and reproductive cancers. Eliminate as much plastic from your life as you can by choosing glass or stainless steel containers instead, and wax paper, cellophane, or parchment for wrapping foods.

One of the greatest imbalances for our reproductive systems is our diminished link with nature. A lack of connection with the natural world can cause a dissociation from the rhythms of earth and sky, thus creating glandular disharmony. Additionally, human interference with Earth's natural rhythms directly interferes with our own. Pollutants, radiation from microwaves, cell towers, and phones, computers, and fluorescent lighting all disrupt intracellular communication and can disrupt endocrine balance.

The Female Reproductive System

The female reproductive cycle reflects the lunar cycle and is often timed with it, as a twenty-eight to thirty-five-day menstrual cycle, resulting in approximately thirteen moons per year. A woman's body is defined by breasts, ovaries, fallopian tubes, uterus, vagina, and clitoris (see diagram 4, page 144). Each menstrual cycle begins when the last one has ended, as the brain senses low levels of estrogen in the blood and sends a message to the pituitary gland to release FSH, which travels through the bloodstream to stimulate the ovaries to develop eggs in their follicles. As an egg develops, it makes estrogen, causing estrogen levels to rise. The developing egg keeps maturing while several others die off and turn into surrounding ovarian tissue. By about day fourteen, there is enough estrogen in the body to trigger the pituitary to release LH, which causes more blood to circulate into the ovaries, and, with the help of enzymes, the mature egg is liberated from its follicle in ovulation. The empty follicle forms the corpus luteum, which makes progesterone to prepare the uterus for implantation, maintain a pregnancy, and promote breast-milk production. Without fertilization of the egg, now waiting in the fallopian tube for a swimming sperm, the corpus luteum stops making progesterone, and menstruation occurs.

Adolescence

During adolescence, hormone production and secretion increases at an unsteady rate. "Hormone" comes from the Greek *hormon,* "to urge on; to excite" — hormones are stimulating! As the body accommodates this new reality, physical and psychological changes occur that some parents refer to as the "terrible teens." While this spurt of life-force may feel raging to some, it's exciting, highly energetic, and liberating. Such energy can be channeled constructively or destructively, though in industrialized societies, the inherent innovation and creativity of teenagers too often goes unnoticed or unnourished. Many girls now begin puberty as early as age nine; some of this due to exposure to steroid hormones in foods (especially animal products pumped with growth hormones), drugs, and municipal water systems, along with poor diet and lack of exercise.

The female reproductive system is very intricate and needs excellent nourishment to develop. Estrogen (of which there are many kinds), is responsible for growth of the endometrium (uterine lining), relaxes blood vessel walls, improves circulation, repairs cell tissue, stimulates secretions of the cervix, imparts sex characteristics, retains bone calcium, and uplifts emotions — a hormone of outward-moving energy. Progesterone prepares for and supports pregnancy (cell building) and lactation, organizes cells, and calms sexual drive — a hormone of inward-moving energy. Follicle-stimulating hormone (FSH) is produced for the growth and development of the follicle, wherein the egg develops while in the ovary. Luteinizing hormone (LH) controls the production of estrogens and androgens (the more "masculine" sex characteristics). Prolactin initiates and maintains the flow of breast milk, and can suppress ovary function during lactation. In adolescence, hormonal response is developing, so there's a need to nourish and strengthen the endocrine glands in general, and to attend to the liver, which stores and releases excess hormones in particular.

Herbs and foods for building glandular strength include burdock root, astragalus, rehmannia root, nettle, kelp, wild yam, alfalfa, red raspberry leaf, vitex (*Vitex agnus castus*), hops, dong quai, super-greens (the grasses, algae, spirulina), molasses, bee pollen, royal jelly, all squashes, coconut, flaxseed, pumpkin seed, sesame seed, fish, olive oil, root vegetables, nuts and seeds, leafy greens, and whole grains.

Limit cane sugar and refined foods such as white bread and pastries in the diet as much as possible; save sodas for special occasions and drink plenty of water and fresh-squeezed juices. If you wish to consume animal products, be sure they're organic and free of growth hormones and antibiotics.

Make a pot of this tea and drink it throughout the day to acquire trace minerals:

Vita-Mins Tea

2 parts each: nettle leaf, red raspberry leaf, oatstraw, gotu-kola, and alfalfa

1 part each: calendula flower, rosehip, horsetail, peppermint, and licorice root

Steep, covered, at least 20 minutes (the longer the better) and drink throughout the day.

Today, many adolescents spend time intimately exposed to electromagnetic radiation emitted by cell or portable phones, computers, cordless phones, and other electronic equipment. Studies have shown that such exposure disrupts cellular communication within the brain and has a direct effect on glandular development — so be aware and limit exposure time to electromagnetic devices as much as possible. Kombu seaweed and personalized flower-remedy combinations can help mitigate some of the effects of exposure.

Caring for our liver (which must process excess and uneven hormone loads) will calm emotions and clear the skin. Herbs like dandelion, Oregon grape, wild yam, yellow dock, burdock, birch bark, sassafras, sarsaparilla, garlic, cayenne, and citrus are very helpful (see chapter three for teas and tinctures). Also GLA (gamma linolenic acid), found in oils of borage, evening primrose, and black currant, help regulate prostaglandin production. Prostaglandins are hormone-like substances that mediate a range of functions, such as control of blood pressure, contraction of smooth muscle, and modulation of inflammation; their excess in the bloodstream results in menstrual discomfort, mood swings, and cramps.

De-cramp Decoction

2 parts cramp bark or black haw (*Viburnum prunifolium*)
1 part each: cinnamon bark, wild yam, and ginger

Simmer, covered, 20 minutes, take off heat and add ½ part lobelia (or tincture of lobelia), and steep another 5 minutes before pouring off. Sweeten with molasses or honey as desired. Alternatively, licorice root or stevia leaf can be added.

Drink half a cup of the above tea 2 to 3 times a day during the week before menses. When cramping occurs, drink ¼ cup every 15 minutes. Ginger and hops compresses, or alternating hot and cold packs on the lower belly, also provide relief. Rubbing essential oils of lavender, sweet marjoram, or chamomile on the lower torso can also help, especially before bed. Eat plenty of calcium- and magnesium-rich foods and juices.

Herbs for amenorrhea (absent or delayed menses) can be divided into two groups. One group of herbs *moves and directs stagnant blood* from the liver; these are rue, dong quai, blue cohosh, ginger, mugwort, Roman chamomile, or pennyroyal leaf, along with foods that stimulate the liver. The other group addresses *blood deficiency*: black cohosh, yarrow, vitex, dong quai, codonopsis, and parsley, plus soft-cooked neutral foods that nourish the spleen (especially soups and cooked vegetables and whole grains). The GLA in evening oils of primrose, borage, or black currant, along with essential oils of fennel or clary sage, minerals, plus protein and iron-rich foods, also helps support menses. If stress is the cause of blood stagnation, rest and bodywork will often bring on menses. If bleeding halts abruptly mid-menses, yogic inversion poses such as shoulder stands can help bleeding to resume. Note that strong alkaloids in coffee and black tea can stimulate the start of menses if a stagnant liver is the issue. With constant use, however, they can lead to liver stagnation, disrupting menses and depleting mineral stores, which causes blood deficiency. It's far better to build blood with nettle during the entire menstrual cycle.

Herbs for menorrhagia (excessive menstrual bleeding) include yarrow, red raspberry, red rose petal(*Rosa* spp.), shepherd's purse (*Capsella bursa-pastoris*), lady's mantle (*Alchemilla vulgaris*), white oak bark, cayenne, and kelp. Make sure you get enough iron from nettles, alfalfa, cherries, figs, apricots, and root vegetables. Avoid caffeine and non-organic animal products. Use the following tea to halt excessive bleeding:

Ease the Flow Tea

2 parts each: shepherd's purse and red raspberry

1 part each: sage, rose hip, red rose petal, and yarrow

Tincture of white oak bark can be added to every cup of tea to further increase its styptic quality. Powdered sap of dragon blood plant (Croton lechleri) can be taken in severe cases.

Child-bearing Years – From Flower to Fruit

The phase between adolescence and menopause is a time of birthing, mothering, and nurturing whether creating a family, creating a business, or both! It's a time of building one's life and community — the waxing-to-full-moon stage during which it's highly beneficial for a woman to fortify and support her reproductive system.

In comparison to men, women may feel their reproductive parts are complicated and beset with challenges, but a plethora of herbs are available. Listen to your body when it speaks, by consulting your inner physician. The interrelationship between hormones, organs, and emotional and spiritual development is unique for each woman and is strongly influenced by her relationship with her own body. Feeling at home and comfortable with your body is part of cultivating self-love and reverence for the unique person you are. Feeling good about ourselves and our lives does much to balance hormones!

The uterus is the strongest muscle in the female body, and, like the moon, it goes through its monthly waxing and waning phases that require key nutrients. Many of the premenstrual cravings women have are nutrient related — even dark chocolate is sought after because of its relatively high (per weight) magnesium and iron content, not to mention its endorphins. Ms. Uterus is like an Olympic athlete gearing up for the big event every month — so support her with whole foods high in the nutrients she needs. Remember that this muscle is the throne of your creative power, on which sit the divine gifts (symbolized by your eggs) that you bring into fruition by expressing your authentic self. Honor your cycle and the physiology that dances it!

Herbs and foods to tone and strengthen the uterus: black cohosh, partridge berry (*Michella repens*), dong quai, ginger, licorice, false unicorn root (*Chamaelirium luteum*), motherwort, nettle, strawberry, blackberry, and raspberry leaves. These herbs can be used for long periods of time, but note that using black cohosh or dong quai during menses will encourage heavier bleeding. Be sure your diet provides plenty of high-quality plant protein and iron-rich foods. Stimulate the pelvic area with alternate hot and cold sitz baths, dancing, sexual activity, deep breathing, Kegel exercises (squeezing and releasing the perineum as if to stop urination), aerobic exercise, yoga (especially inversion postures), and massage.

Menstruation and ovulation are dependent upon hormonal signals influenced by the brain and nervous system. Therefore, emotions, the connection with one's inner nature and the natural world, combined with stress, together strongly influence the balance of chemical signals. If you're going through difficult times, cleansing, in athletic training, or moving through big changes, you may find your cycle being disrupted or skipped altogether. Plants have their own hormonal system. They don't have estrogen and progesterone exactly like ours, but they do have phytoestrogens or steroidal compounds that are compatible with the human body, and we can use those compounds as building blocks to formulate our own steroidal hormones. The natural wisdom of our body defines how the unique synergistic interaction between plant and person affects each of us. This is why women's bodies differ in their response to various plant steroids. Remember, hormones are communicators, and how each person communicates internally does vary. That said, there are classic formulas for balancing the female cycle that have proven themselves effective.

Herbs and foods that promote hormonal balance by providing precursors to human hormone production are alfalfa, black cohosh, black haw, dong quai, licorice, asparagus root / Shatavari (*Asparagus racemosus*), vitex, wild yam, blessed thistle (*Cnicus benedictus*), fennel, hops, soy, pomegranate, saw palmetto (*Serenoa repens*), false unicorn root and maca root. Vitamin E-rich foods such as wheat germ, avocados, coconut, macadamia nut, olive oil, soy, and most nuts and seeds help. Vitamin E assists the liver in breaking down excess estrogen and normalizing hormones in general. The following formula addresses female hormone balance.

Female Balance – Wild Woman Tincture

3 parts each: dong quai, vitex (chaste tree), and partridge berry

2 parts each: wild yam, black cohosh, American ginseng, and hops

1 part each: licorice, juniper berry, and damiana

If you're accustomed to delayed menses, add 1 part yarrow as well. This is best taken as a tincture. Take 40 drops 3 times a day starting about 2 days after the end of menses until the start of menses, unless you're trying to become pregnant, in which case stop the tincture at ovulation. This tincture can be taken for months to balance irregularities, or just used during specific months that you know might be hormonally challenged.

Pregnancy

Bringing a new life into the world celebrates a time of reverence and awe. Though it is the mother who directly experiences the miracle of gestation, everyone involved can be present in the process with willingness, understanding, and love — all essential to the well-being of the child. What mom eats and drinks will construct the child's body. The energies of a mother's thoughts and feelings and of those around her will influence the child, just as our thoughts and feelings affect our own cells. Pregnancy is a time to discover the power and support of "gentle" herbs and foods! It is a time to build and tone the body and to balance feeding oneself while feeding the developing child within — and to do this without overburdening the heart, circulatory system, and other organs. It's wise to cleanse the colon, liver, and kidneys *before* conception, and eat nutritious *organic* foods with plenty of B vitamins (especially folate / folic acid) and omega-3 oils, since nerve-sheath development in the brain and spinal cord are particularly crucial in the first six weeks of life.

Easily absorbed, high-quality super-foods such as alfalfa, wheat-grass, chlorella, spirulina, blue-green algae, kelp, barley, and oat grasses will provide vitamins and minerals — especially the B's and iron. Limit consumption of fish, since mercury, present in all fish, is damaging to a fetus. Pregnancy is not the time for heavy detoxification programs, but minor, supervised cleansing of the bowel and liver with foods, juices, and tonic herbs can be carried out if necessary. Suitable and safe cleansing herbs, like dandelion, milk thistle, burdock, and chicory can be taken for the liver, which has a tendency to become overworked, overheated, and congested with all the extra hormonal commitments it has to cope with.

There are herbs that support both mother and baby by toning and strengthening the uterus and providing nutrients: wild yam, nettles, lady's mantle, yellow dock, chickweed, alfalfa, red raspberry leaves, dandelion root and leaves, and partridgeberry after the sixth month. For more in-depth information, see the references section for some excellent herb books dedicated to women's health.

A common occurrence in the first few weeks of pregnancy is morning sickness, often caused by massive changes in hormone levels combined with low blood sugar and even low blood pressure. Useful herbs for morning sickness include wild yam, dandelion, ginger, vitex, peppermint, chamomile, and hops. Ginger is safe to take, but keep quantities moderate. To reduce symptoms, keep a few crackers by the bedside to eat before rising in the morning. To prevent heartburn, eat small meals and chew well. Add digestive herbs such as anise, caraway, fennel, peppermint, spearmint, meadowsweet, fenugreek, cinnamon, and lavender to your food, or take as a tea after meals.

To curb constipation try carob, slippery elm, flaxseed, psyllium, licorice, burdock, aloe vera, yogurt, sauerkraut, miso, yellow dock, prune juice, watermelon, and triphala or Turkey rhubarb; also be sure to consume plenty of fiber and water. Supplemental acidophilus is very helpful and supports the immune system, while magnesium supports the heart and relaxes the intestines.

Eating organically is of prime importance, since pesticides are neurotoxins and can influence brain development. While in the womb, a baby is defenseless — avoid exposure to environmental toxins.

Some herbs should not be ingested during pregnancy, especially in the first three months, before the placenta has fully formed. Herbs rich in alkaloids, for example, can act as uterine stimulants and trigger miscarriage: barberry root, coffee, poke root (*Phytolacca americana*), goldenseal, dong quai, juniper, black cohosh, nutmeg, mace, yarrow, angelica, motherwort, pennyroyal, thuja, rue, mistletoe, lobelia, yarrow, sage, wormwood, comfrey, and coltsfoot. Partridgeberry can be taken pre-conception and then again after the sixth month of pregnancy.

Herbs safe to use should you have an infection are echinacea in moderate amounts, and elderberry. Herbs such as elderflower and berry, mullein, red raspberry, cleavers, chickweed, and oatstraw are also safe. Listen to your body and follow your intuition — if you feel uneasy about taking an herb or food, don't consume it. Most of your medicine can come from your meals: eating all the colors of the rainbow gives a full spectrum of nutrients! To reduce water retention, nettles, melons, dandelion, and cucumber are effective diuretics. For a refreshing diuretic drink, peel and chop a whole cucumber and puree in the blender with some spring water and a dash of fresh mint. Brewer's yeast is a good way to get folic acid, along with super-greens, whole grains, strawberries (organic only!), and prenatal vitamins.

Threat of Miscarriage

Where there is spot bleeding and the threat of miscarriage, inform your midwife and / or physician immediately. Sometimes miscarriage is the body's natural response to specific situations, and in such circumstances, no herbal remedy will oppose it. Threat of miscarriage can, however, also be triggered by stress, trauma, inadequate diet, or hormonal imbalance, in which case herbs can provide extra strength or help calm muscles to avoid it. Bed rest and removal of stress factors are most important, then follow with herbs traditionally used to prevent miscarriage: black haw, cramp bark, false unicorn root, lobelia, and wild yam. These are antispasmodic and relaxing for the uterine muscles and nerves. Where there is threat of miscarriage, make the following tincture before or at the start of pregnancy, or prepare as a decoction when needed, adding lobelia and raspberry leaf to steep after simmering the roots.

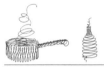

Baby Be Formula

2 parts cramp bark, black haw root bark and false unicorn root

1 part each: red raspberry leaf (add after decocting above roots)

½ part each: lobelia

While in a reclined position, drink half a cup every half hour until the bleeding stops, then every waking hour for a day. Continue to drink half a cup 3 times a day for the next 7 – 14 days. If taking as a tincture, add a half teaspoon of tincture to warm water or tea (for example, tea of shepherd's purse and / or yarrow to further arrest bleeding). In addition, acupuncture and taking 800iu of mixed-tocopherol Vitamin E can also help.

Birthing

In the last four weeks of pregnancy, prepare the whole body for labor by using a birthing tincture such as:

Beautiful Birth Tincture

Equal parts: partridgeberry, red raspberry, blessed thistle, black cohosh root, pennyroyal leaf, and false unicorn root

½ part lobelia

Prepared as a tincture or strong tea steeped overnight and brought to a boil in the morning, this formula gives elasticity to the pelvic and vaginal areas, strengthening and toning the reproductive system for a smooth delivery. Take 20 – 40 drops of the tincture twice a day or sip two cups of tea throughout the day. Mist your space with calming floral waters like lavender or rose.

To stimulate labor, try a dropper-full of blue cohosh tincture in ginger tea every hour. Homeopathic *caulophyllum* (200c) can also promote contractions, as can Beth root / white trillium root (*Trillium erectum*).

During birth, parsley root, pennyroyal, blue cohosh, black cohosh, dong quai, cotton root (*Gossypium herbaceum*), and rue will help promote contractions, while lobelia will help dilate the cervix. After birthing, tincture of elecampane or blue cohosh can aid in release of the placenta. Soaking in a slightly warm sitz bath of red rose petals, red hibiscus flowers, and yarrow flowers will alleviate bleeding and heal tissues of the vagina and labia, as can tincture of witch hazel. Sometimes the uterus becomes prolapsed after birth, in which case toning herbs such as partridge berry, hibiscus flower, and yarrow can be taken as tea. Relaxing on a slant-board for ten minutes twice a day, or lying in bed with a pillow under your hips and massaging the lower belly with strong upward strokes, can help the uterus reposition itself. To restore your vitality, use herbs such as lady's mantle, vitex, licorice, eleuthero, nettle, comfrey leaf, oatstraw, and chamomile.

It is best for a baby to be breast-fed just after delivery, when the clear colostrum is present (it lasts about two days). Breast milk is the richest source of food for your baby, and helps build a strong immune system immediately. For breast-feeding use *galactagogues,* herbs that promote milk flow. A nice combination is the following:

Mama's Milk Tea

Equal parts: partridge berry herb, fennel seed, nettle leaf, blessed thistle leaf, marshmallow root, milky oatstraw tops, and rose petals

Put 4 tablespoons of herb mixture into a quart of cold water. Slowly bring to a boil, remove from heat, cover, and steep for 15 – 20 minutes.
Drink 4 cups of this tea daily. It will help restore your strength and promote a good supply of nutritious milk for your baby. If you're suffering severe depletion or night sweats, tincture of vitex (20 drops per cup of tea) can be added to help balance hormones.

Other galactagogues are milk thistle, fenugreek seed, caraway seed, motherwort, vervain, and hops. For drying up breast milk once weaning has ensued, use sage, large amounts of parsley, shepherd's purse or wormwood tea, and other bitter or astringent herbs. The milk will slowly become bitter as productivity wanes, and your baby will reject it simultaneously over several days — a gentle way to handle a sometimes difficult transition.

Menopause – Moon Pause

Childhood, adolescence, childbearing… and now a new cycle begins. Menopause is a time of gathering one's wisdom and finding new ways of harnessing and using one's creativity and power — *yes!* It's also a big metamorphosis and very personal experience. Power surges indicate that it's time to manage one's life differently. The perimenopause (premenopausal phase) can begin anywhere between the ages thirty-seven to fifty, and moving through menopause can last from two to ten years.

How you experience menopause depends partly on your expression of feelings and needs, your emotional views regarding this physical change, and your ideas about aging. Keep in mind that hereditary factors and the intricacies of your body chemistry play a role. No two women are alike in how they experience menopause, and, no matter what, one must work with one's self.

Women with more stress in their lives may experience more of the possible symptoms: hot flashes, insomnia, night sweats, depression, and vaginal dryness. How you've handled your body in previous years will influence your menopause. Any accumulated and unattended health issues, emotional patterns, and toxic buildup come to the fore — sometimes rather vehemently. Nothing eases endocrine changes and balances the body more than basic cleansing, rest, sound nutrition, and exercise.

Often, menopausal symptoms are worsened by the exhaustion or depletion of adrenal glands and kidneys. Avoiding substances that exaggerate this condition (sugar, caffeine, alcohol, fried foods, cold foods, and uncultured dairy) is important! Foods and herbs that nourish, moisten, and strengthen the kidneys (see previous chapter) are necessary, especially if you're very active or currently cleansing.

Not all women suffer: some have difficult symptoms, some have minor symptoms, and others hardly notice any changes at all. Multitudes of plant allies can assist women during this time. Excellent books are available covering this subject (see references).

Many herbal formulas use some combination of dong quai, red clover, black cohosh, vitex or wild yam, plus or minus various herbs that calm nerves, balance liver (moods and hot flashes) and kidneys (water retention and fear of change) while assisting the heart. These formulas work well when taken consistently, 30 – 60 drops (dosage depends on body weight and sensitivity), three times a day, six days a week, for three months, along with the Revitalizing Diet (chapter one) and daily exercise of some kind. Many women prefer to take isoflavone capsules (usually concentrated from soy — remember, *all* beans have phytoestrogens), or concentrated black cohosh or red clover supplements, and some use all-natural plant sterol creams, or a combination of these remedies. Tune in to what intuitively attracts you and start with that.

Manageable Menopause

2 parts each: dong quai, vitex, black cohosh, and wild yam

1 part each: red clover, hawthorn berry, and ashwaganda root

½ part each: licorice and damiana

Prepare as a decoction and drink 3 – 5 cups a day, or make as a tincture and take 2 – 4 teaspoons (depending on body weight and metabolism) per day; mix into hot water or tea to allow the alcohol to dissipate.

The above can be taken along with the following supportive tea:

Feminine Flourish Tea

2 parts each: alfalfa, red clover flowers, nettle leaf, and lemon verbena

1 part each: blessed thistle, oatstraw, partridge berry herb, calendula flower, red raspberry leaf, and rose petals

½ part each: damiana and motherwort

Vitex berries (chaste tree berry) assist the pituitary in balancing secretions, and can be included as a daily tonic. Dandelion, sarsaparilla, and sassafras balance the endocrine system through action of the liver. Black cohosh, red clover, maca root, turmeric and sage leaf will reduce severity and frequency of hot flashes, while herbs such as rehmannia root support the kidneys. Hot flashes are greatly influenced by overall liver health. Avoid "hot" foods that create excess heat in the body such as (you guessed it!) coffee, black tea, alcohol, recreational drugs, chocolate, refined sugars, saturated and cooked fats, and cooked hot spices. A congested liver cannot effectively deal with hormonal tidal waves!

Liver cleansing using supporting herbs (see chapter three) will free the liver to process hormones more efficiently. Ease hot flashes by increasing calcium, taking 800iu mixed-tocopherol vitamin E, drinking *lots of water,* and increasing your electrolyte intake. Calcium and magnesium will aid the heart, along with herbs that calm and protect it, such as hawthorn berry, motherwort, rose petals, linden flower, and borage, plus diuretic herbs and foods. Aromatherapy using rose hydrosol spray is very calming to the heart.

Vaginal dryness often accompanies the menopausal process, but can be helped by:

Get Juicy Tea

Equal parts: red clover, red raspberry leaf, and rose hips

½ **part** damiana

Prepare as a tea and drink throughout the day.

Get Juicy Tincture

1 part milky oat grass tops tinctured in glycerin

1 part damiana tinctured in alcohol

plus **one drop** of pure rose oil (or several drops of rose water if you don't have the oil)

Keep this tincture by the bedside and take 1 – 2 droppers full each morning and evening:

Additionally, vitamin E, super-greens, omega-3 oils, whole soybeans, maca root, asparagus root-Shatavari, licorice, and alfalfa grass and sprouts help. The vaginal lining can be topically nourished with aloe vera gel, or a combination of wild yam, calendula, comfrey, and St. John's wort extracted in olive oil. Aromatherapy oils used in massage, or body lotion of clary sage, rose geranium, and orange are balancing.

Nerves often need extra support with spirulina or blue-green algae, B vitamin foods, baths, beach walks, and a good bedtime tea:

 ## Bedtime is Beautiful Tea

Equal parts: chamomile, any mint, lemon balm, skullcap, passionflower, lavender flower, and valerian root or blue vervain flowering tops

St. John's wort can be added to any formula to address depressive tendencies. Severe depression, however, warrants professional care.

Flower remedies offer much during a time of menopausal change and can be taken liberally! In addition, use adrenal-support herbs such as eleuthero, American ginseng, astragalus, flax, medicinal mushrooms, codonopsis root, evening primrose, borage, nettle, licorice, ashwaganda, bee pollen, and royal jelly.

Help For Common Ailments

Endometriosis

Endometriosis ensues when the uterine lining (endometrium) produces small nests of cells that migrate to sites outside the uterus, such as the fallopian tubes, ovaries, bladder, and other areas in the pelvic cavity (or, rarely, outside the pelvic cavity). During the menstrual cycle, these pieces of endometrium respond to progesterone by thickening in post-ovulation as the uterus does, thus causing discomfort and heavy bleeding at menses. Endometriosis is the most common source of infertility. It is often caused by over-secretion of estrogen, incomplete menstrual cycles, lack of circulation to the pelvic cavity, animal steroids in food, xenoestrogens (estrogen-mimicking compounds) present in food and drink containers and as byproducts of the plastic industry, and possibly an under-functioning immune system.

Natural treatment of endometriosis includes avoiding the use of plastics and foods that tend to raise estrogen levels, such as animal products, wheat, potato (nightshades in general), yam, soy, hops (beer), coffee, tea, and chocolate. Herbs with estrogenic effect, such as red clover, fennel, pomegranate, and blessed thistle, should be reduced, though more often these can have a regulating effect. Treating the liver is key, as well as cleansing the bowel entirely. Blood-cleansing and moving herbs such as Oregon grape, dong quai, turmeric, blue cohosh, chaparral, pau d'arco, and goldenseal are very effective. Vitex, white peony root (*Paeonia officialis, P. albiflora*), wild yam, vitamin E, and GLA will help restore hormonal balance. Shiitake, maitake, and reishi mushrooms, green tea, and neem leaf serve to inhibit abnormal tissue growth. Don't forget castor-oil packs, sitz baths, and hot / cold showers to increase circulation to your pelvic area. Flower remedies, massage, acupressure, visualization, and paying attention to your dreams can also help.

Premenstrual Tension (PMT)

Premenstrual tension is characterized by irritability, mood swings, sugar cravings, and generally feeling overwhelmed; all of these are symptoms connected with stagnant liver energy, which is often the cause of PMT! Liver-cleansing herbs and even a liver flush can help. Eat lightly (veggie juices are great), increase your antioxidants, *exercise*, rest, relax, and do fun things for yourself (humorous movies are a great aid).

Often, premenstrual tension is an expression of built-up resentment over *not doing what really inspires you*. Honoring the reproductive cycle is honoring yourself and your true needs. Irritability and sugar cravings are also hallmarks of mineral deficiency, especially iron. Be sure your diet is rich in raw and lightly steamed greens, sea vegetables, vegetable juices, and superfoods. Drink iron-rich tea or take an iron tonic (see chapter four).

All women produce small amounts of testosterone. There is a slight (though noticeable, once you tune in to it) testosterone surge just about two days before menses. For many women this results in a surge of energy that needs outlet in some constructive way — *physically* moving this energy is important! Eat whole grains, vegetables, and fruits, but drop the fats, the dairy (soft-cooked eggs are fine), fried, refined, and sugary foods. Add lecithin, seaweed, and brewer's yeast to your diet. Hormone-balancing herbs, flower remedies, and essential oils of rose geranium, clary sage, petigrain, and rose are helpful. If PMT has always been a major challenge, it's time to seriously consider bowel and liver cleansing to free the liver of its load and bring the body back to balance.

Herbs that help support the body during the menstrual cycle: eleuthero, fo-ti / He Shou Wu, dong quai, American ginseng, ashwaganda, vitex, black cohosh, red raspberry, dandelion root, nettle leaf, suma, maca root, rehmannia root, wild yam, astragalus, holy basil / tulsi, asparagus root / Shatavari, damiana and foods containing omega-3 oils. Nurture the nervous system with herbs like motherwort, lemon balm, Roman chamomile, lavender, oatstraw, hops, blue vervain, and skullcap — and don't forget the kidney herbs to reduce water retention!

Ovarian Cysts

An ovarian cyst is a sac — often filled with fluid or semisolid material — that develops in or on the ovary. It may come and go or be a symptom of disease, so it's important to have it checked by a doctor. Most ovarian cysts are benign and can be reduced or dissolved altogether by undertaking a healing regime that includes bowel cleansing, liver flushes, castor oil packs, and the use of dissolving herbs such as Oregon grape root, barberry, goldenseal, red root, and yerba mansa (*Anemopsis californica*).

Vaginal Yeast Infections

Yeast infections (candida overgrowth) are uncomfortable and can become chronic, especially if there has been long-standing digestive insufficiency or suppression of the immune system. Candida overgrowth causes itching of the vagina and / or anus and presents a strong-smelling, cottage cheese-like vaginal discharge. A pap smear can be taken to confirm whether the discharge is candida, since some STDs (sexually transmitted diseases) also result in thick, odoriferous discharges. Treatment of candida overgrowth requires an alkaline diet (vegetables, whole grains, and mostly plant protein), and eliminating sweets, including alcohol, foods containing yeast, and most fruits until alkalinity is restored. A bowel cleanse that includes bentonite clay will help pull excess yeast off the intestinal lining.

Herbs such as sage, red raspberry leaf, mullein, echinacea, myrrh, pau d'arco, thyme, thuja, black walnut, garlic, wormwood, Oregon grape root, and goldenseal all fight fungus when taken as teas, tinctures, capsules, or in a douche. Essential oils of oregano, rosemary, cinnamon, and tea tree taken internally in small amounts can be very effective (be sure to have high-quality oils). Essential oils or fresh herbs can also be used in a warm sitz bath or vaginal steam (like a facial steam, except you kneel or crouch over the bowl and cover your legs with a blanket. GSE (grapefruit-seed extract) is effective in liquid form (10 – 15 drops in water two to three times daily) or in capsules. Taking probiotics morning and evening will re-establish flora in the colon, which is pressing against the vagina. A *vaginal bolus* or *pessary* is an herb-and-oil paste formed to fit into the vagina like a tampon. It's easily made by mixing softened coconut oil into the following:

Vaginal Bolus

Use finely powdered and sieved herbs only.

3 parts slippery elm

1 part each: black walnut hull, myrrh, pau d'arco

½ part goldenseal (barberry root bark or Oregon grape root bark can be substituted).

Several drops of lavender oil and tea tree oil

Make a bolus by mixing enough softened coconut oil into herb mixture to form a thick paste, then shape, and cool in the refrigerator. When you want to use one, take one out of the refrigerator and briefly warm between your fingers before inserting it. You might wish to use a bit of olive oil to lubricate the area of insertion first. Your body temperature will cause the coconut oil to melt and the herbs to disperse. Whether you use a bolus day or night, wear a panty liner.

A very simplified version of the bolus:

Lightly drizzle an organic cotton tampon with tea tree oil, then dip or roll it in castor oil (just enough to cover) before inserting into your vagina.

Remember to notice how your lifestyle choices may be stressing you, and whether you've honored your personal boundaries — where you are and another person begins — in your relationships. Personal stress or anxiety is often a factor in candida overgrowth, so support your nervous system with strengthening and calming nervines (see chapter eight). Extreme temperature change, especially to cool, damp climates, or exposure to chemicals, can alter blood pH and create a more hospitable environment for yeast to grow. Sunshine and fresh air can make the difference!

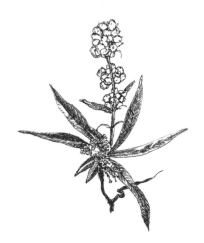

The Male Reproductive System

There are no "guy-necologists" to say so, but men have reproductive cycles too! The more a man becomes aware of his subtle internal rhythms, the better he can manage his energies and use his creative potential. Herbs for the male system are nearly the same as those for the female — after all, male development in the embryo is similar. The prostate is like the male "uterus," since it is an organ of nourishment that is dependent upon the endocrine system. The testicles are similar to "ovaries," and are likewise governed by the pituitary gland. The testes produce both testosterone and estrogen. For an in-depth and humorous account of herbal help for the male system, both men and women are referred to James Green's *Male Herbal*.

Adolescent Males

Adolescent males require the same liver-cleansing, plus high mineral herbs and wholesome diet, required for female adolescents. The liver must process the influx of hormones, whose side effects, such as acne, are usually a result of congested liver and bowels. Keep elimination channels open with plenty of fresh fruits and vegetables. Enjoy vigorous physical exercise, which will clear your skin and build your lungs! If there are mood swings, problems with concentration, and nervous stress, take omega-3 essential fatty acids, found in fish and many nuts and seeds like borage, coconut, flax, hemp, macadamia nut, wheat germ, poppy, and pumpkinseed. Appropriate nervines, as discussed in the following chapter, can help reduce nervous tension.

Male Hormones

For balancing the male hormone system, many of the same female-balancing hormones can be used, but use vitex, hops, and dong quai only for short periods of time (not more than two weeks) to address current issues. Herbs more specific to male hormonal balance are saw palmetto, pygeum bark (*Prunus Africana*), puncture vine (*Tribulis terrestris*), nettle root, garlic, gingko, goat weed (*Epimedium grandiflorum*), and all *panax* (Chinese, Korean, American) gingsengs. Foods such as pumpkin seeds, sunflower seeds, tomatoes, sea vegetables, sprouts, and leafy greens all support the prostate gland, as they are high in zinc and other trace minerals.

The maca root of Peru has long been touted for male virility; actually, it's good for both men and women, since it helps the body adapt to change and supports our adrenal glands, which influence hormone production. Studies have shown that maca root can increase sperm viability and motility. Maca is nutritive, and can be purchased as a pleasant-tasting powder to add to smoothies or cereal. Strengthen your system with the following:

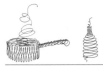

Mega-Male Formula

2 parts each: American ginseng, eleuthero, sarsaparilla, and saw palmetto
1 part each: Chinese or Korean ginseng, wild yam, licorice, Fo-ti (He shou wu), ginger or prickly ash bark, hawthorn berry, and star anise

Simmer as a decoction or make into a tincture. As a tonic, take 2 – 3 cups a day as a tea, or 2 – 3 teaspoons a day in tincture form, for 6 days a week.

Other good herbs for maintenance include white pond lily, figwort, nettle, Oregon grape, gravel root, oatstraw, damiana, marshmallow, mullein, juniper, dandelion, and suma. Notice there are quite a few kidney herbs; keeping the kidneys clear and flowing is crucial for the male genital system, particularly the prostate. The prostate gland can be massaged gently through the perineum to prevent stagnation of fluids. Also, Kegel exercises are as great for men as they are for women. The exercises involve the squeezing and pulling up action required to flex (squeeze) the muscle that's activated when finishing urination. Like the female reproductive system, the male system benefits greatly by cleansing the bowel, liver, and kidneys, and eliminating unnecessary weight. Many problems such as infertility and erectile dysfunction arise from a stressful lifestyle, unexpressed emotional needs, poor nutrition, and lack of exercise or oxygen in general. Take the time to address these issues first before embarking on more involved and / or expensive treatments.

To increase sexual energy, think blood flow to the genitals. For this, such herbs as cayenne, damiana, dong quai, kola nut, and yohimbe bark (*Pausinystalia yohimbe*) are very effective. Yohimbe is a strong circulatory stimulant, so it's best used in small doses as desired; it is not a long-term tonic herb. Keeping genitals cool is important as well; it's best to take a brief cool shower after a hot tub, and cool showers are a good idea if one has driven a vehicle, biked, or sun-bathed for prolonged periods. Alternating hot and cold sitz baths are also effective for stimulating pelvic circulation. Alcohol and cannabis will decrease libido when used consistently or in high dosages.

Help for Common Ailments

Benign Prostate Hypertrophy (BPH)

Benign prostate hypertrophy is swelling of the prostate gland, which compresses and pinches off the urethra, constricting the flow of urine. Nonmalignant enlargement of the prostate is often due to excess tissue growth, spurred by steroid-mimicking compounds that are part of industrial and plastic waste, and growth hormones added to animal products. Infrequent ejaculation can exacerbate this condition. The primary symptom is frequent, slow, or painful urination, particularly at night. If unchecked, urination may become more difficult or nearly stop altogether, which is dangerous to both prostate and kidneys. Don't wait for symptoms to become severe — begin by eliminating the consumption of possible contaminants in food and water, and cleansing the bowel to eliminate accumulated toxins. Then embark on kidney cleansing, including hot and cold sitz baths, and follow with tonic herbs: saw palmetto, pygeum, nettle root, teasel root (*Dipsacus sylvestris*), dandelion root, and pumpkinseed, which address this issue specifically. Remember to add cayenne, ginger, or gingko to keep the blood moving, and before long you'll be feeling fit again!

"Manopause"

The change of life for men is also powerful and often happens in their sixth decade, (typically timed with retirement), where there is a shift of energy, focus, and stamina. Sometimes, men become depressed during this shift in identity, which may present itself as difficulty dealing with internal anger, violence, and sadness; unfortunately, lashing out at loved ones or closing off completely may result. It's a good time for a man to take a break and create some retreat time for himself. It's also a good time to reach out and deepen friendships with other men, support shared interests, travel, and play. As responsibilities shift, new creative interests can develop. Cleansing from top to toe (bowels, liver, and kidneys) is highly recommended, and will help clear emotions and enhance self-expression as well.

Maintaining a balanced diet and exercise program is a must. Herbs such as saw palmetto, fo-ti / He Shou Wu, eleuthero, and nettle root and leaf can be taken indefinitely. Sometimes it's helpful to take vitex for a short period. Other herbs and foods that nourish the prostate are partridge berry, red clover, alfalfa, lycopene (a bioflavonoid found in red fruits and vegetables, especially tomatoes), and foods rich in zinc, calcium, and magnesium (pumpkin and sesame seeds, walnuts, almonds, and oats). Take time out for bodywork, connection with nature, fun, personal innovation, and exploring your creativity. Gather the wisdom cultivated over a lifetime and offer it back to the community in ways that bring you joy.

For both women and men, balance of the endocrine system is strongly influenced by the thyroid gland. Therefore this chapter will end with a discussion of the thyroid and its overall importance in glandular health.

Thinking About the Thyroid

The thyroid is located in the front of the neck, just below the larynx or voice box, and sets overall metabolism, thus affecting the functioning of all organs. It consists of two lobes, one on either side of the trachea (windpipe), and regulates the energy level of nearly every cell in the body. The thyroid's function is to produce the hormones T4 (thyroxin), T3 (triiodothyroinine), and calcitonin, which acts in conjunction with parathyroid hormone to regulate calcium balance.

Thyroid hormones are made from tyrosine (an amino acid present in high levels in the mustard family), and iodine (high amounts found in seaweeds). Other important building blocks are vitamins A, C, and E, selenium, zinc, niacin (B3), pyridoxine (B6), and riboflavin (B2). Women have thyroid glands twice the size of men's, and are eight times more likely than men to have hypothyroidism (underproduction of thyroid hormones), four times more likely to have hyperthyroidism (overproduction of thyroid hormones), and twice as likely to suffer thyroid tumors. Thyroid activity is controlled by the release of TSH (thyroid stimulating hormone) from the pituitary gland, which in turn is regulated by the hypothalamus.

Hypothyroidism

Hypothyroidism is a thyroid deficiency that may result in low basal body temperature, sensitivity to cold, decreased libido, depression, difficulty in losing weight, dry skin, headaches, fatigue, lethargy, heavy menses, and recurrent infections. It may be caused by factors such as hormonal change after pregnancy, grief, poor diet, stress, or iodine depletion from constant use (both internally and externally) of fluoridated, chlorinated, or bromated water supplies. It can also be caused by radioactive iodine (Iodine 131) released from nuclear power plants and weapons facilities, or electrical radiation from cell phones, computers, short-wave radios, and satellite dishes (not to mention satellites themselves). Though iodine is easily taken up by the body (in the large intestine and the skin), it is quickly displaced by heavier molecules like chlorine, fluorine, bromine, pesticide residues, and Iodine 131. Pharmaceutical drugs such as aspirin, warfarin (anticoagulants), Prednisone (corticosteriods), Tetracycline, and xenoestrogens all cause our bodies to *excrete* (thus lose) iodine. Ingesting 3 to 5 grams per day of bladderwrack, Kombu or kelp (as sea vegetable, tablet, or tincture) can restore diminished iodine levels to balance with other minerals in the body. Natural sources of iodine include black walnut, garlic, rosemary, nettle leaf and seed, all root vegetables, mustard greens, chard, parsley, spinach, dandelion, and any produce grown with seaweed fertilizer. Some foods depress thyroid activity.

Avoid eating large quantities (especially if raw) of Brussels sprouts, cabbage, broccoli, cauliflower, kale, peanuts, and pine nuts.

Hyperthyroidism

Hyperthyroidism is the condition of above-normal amounts of thyroid hormones circulating in the body. It is characterized by bulging eyes, accelerated pulse, a tendency to profuse sweats, nervous tremors, restlessness, irritability, emaciation, and increased metabolic rate. Often hereditary, it can also be brought on by stress, poor diet, or absorbing too much industrial iodine.

For example, iodine is used as a disinfecting agent in the dairy business, hospitals, and the food industry. Iodized salt was introduced in the USA in 1924 because a large percentage of the population was afflicted with goiter (enlarged thyroid due to inadequate iodine levels, hormonal imbalance, or autoimmune disease). Industrial iodine comes from brine deposits mined in Oklahoma, Chile, and Japan. Since the 1960s, iodine has been added to flour, cereals, and other packaged foods to prevent spoilage. If one has a tendency to hyperthyroidism then it's important to avoid iodized salt and packaged or processed foods, and consume more organic soy beans, broccoli, cauliflower (the family of cruciferous vegetables as listed above), and herbs such as lemon balm, bugleweed, and motherwort, all of which slow the release of TSH and thus thyroid activity.

Malfunction in thyroid-hormone production can also result from selenium deficiency (selenium is needed for one of the amino-acid bonds). Selenium is leached from the body by heavy metals, particularly mercury, and is being depleted from our soils due to the use of chemical fertilizers and pesticides. Selenium supplementation can be helpful (it's a powerful antioxidant as well), but should not exceed 200 micrograms per day. Organic Brazil nuts and mushrooms contain substantial amounts of selenium and are beneficial in replenishing this mineral.

Perhaps the biggest threat to thyroid health is radioactive iodine, which not only displaces natural iodine, but also exposes nearby cells to gamma radiation in the process! The thyroid is where most of our body iodine is stored, but the next major storage areas are the breasts, other reproductive organs, and the lining of the intestines. The intestines alone can efficiently extract 98 percent of the iodine from our food! The rise in reproductive cancers may also be attributed to radioactive iodine, which is released regularly from nuclear power plants (and used in the food-inspection industry) as strontium. So, how do we keep our bodies from drinking radioactive iodine (which, sadly, is everywhere on the globe)? The trick is to consume enough natural iodine and minerals from whole foods, so your body won't be thirsty for them — eat those sea vegetables!

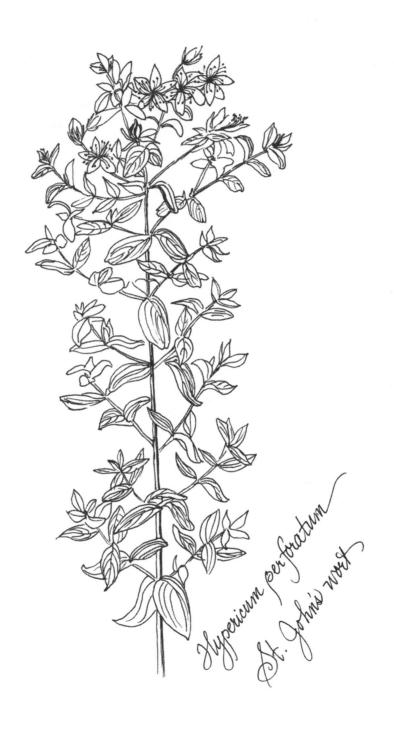

Hypericum perforatum
St. John's wort

Chapter Eight

The Nervous System:
Nerve Cells and Brain

The poppy petals, how calmly they fall.

Etsajin

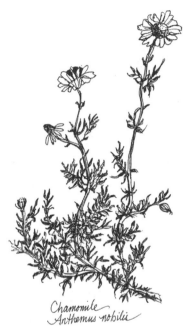

Chamomile
Anthemus nobilii

If we stop to observe, we see that everything in nature is constantly exchanging information. Cells communicate with each other, whether they are microbes in the soil, organisms in water or land, fungal forms, insects, plants, or animals. Everything is busily sending out and receiving signals via chemicals, sound, light, color, sonar, electrical, or other forms of energy exchange. Like a single cell in the universal body, the earth constantly interacts with other planets, stars, and galaxies. In our own body, cells from all tissues and organs "talk" with one another and with their environment. Our nervous system coordinates all communication between our perception of the outside world and the intricacies of our internal environment, creating a feedback loop of information on which cellular decisions are based. It is highly tuned to using both gross and subtle signals to maintain balance or homeostasis between two worlds. Our nervous system reflects the relationship between the physical and psychological aspects of our being, and therefore is always included in any holistic treatment of health imbalances.

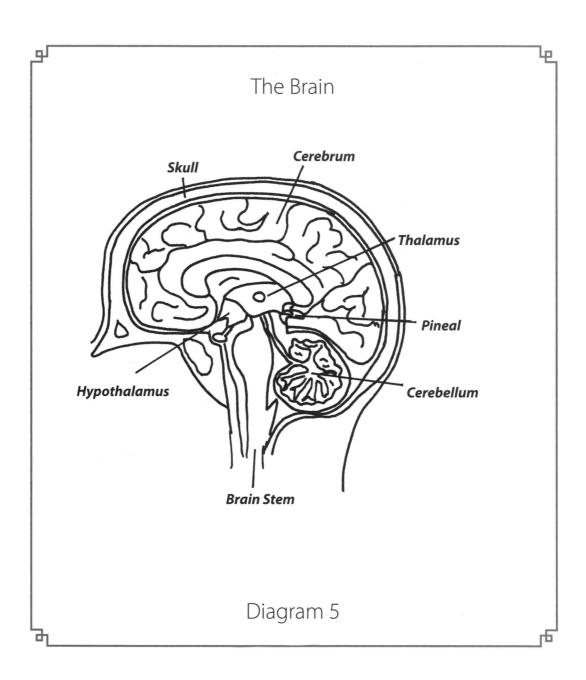

The Brain

Diagram 5

The Nerves

The nervous system is designed to simultaneously gather information about the external environment and our body's internal state by way of its connection with our subtle energy or electromagnetic field. Information is analyzed, initiating appropriate responses aimed at satisfying certain desires, whether survival, pleasure, excitement, internal balance, or avoiding unpleasant negative emotions or pain. Though the cells that make up the nervous system are simple, the system itself is highly complex.

What we call nerves are actually bundles of nerve cells called neurons, which consist of a cell body and a long fiber called an axon. Some axons are very long, running from the spinal cord to the feet! For a message to pass from the spinal cord to a toe, for instance, an electrochemical impulse is sent down the axon toward a receptor; between the two is a synapse or space, over which the impulse must jump with the help of neurotransmitters such as acetylcholine or serotonin. Our nervous system is similar to the electrical wiring of our homes, with our nerve fluid acting as electrical current. Each nerve cell has a protective myelin sheath, just as wires are coated with insulation. When nerve endings get worn out, this sheath starts to fray and the nerve becomes overly sensitive (and we become "frazzled").

Our bodies are indeed electrical, and the nervous system may become overstimulated as an electrical charge builds up over the course of a day. This is especially true if one is treading predominantly on city pavement or synthetic rugs, surrounded by the electrical fields of our homes, lightning storms, radio antennas, cell towers, power lines, and computers. To dissipate the charge we must ground ourselves, as with all electrical systems. The time-honored tradition of walking barefoot on the grass in order to settle down and sleep really does work because it dissipates these excess charges.

Nerves, which affect both our physical and emotional well-being, consist of two major parts: the peripheral nervous system or PNS (cranial and spinal nerves) and the central nervous system or CNS (brain and spinal cord).

The Peripheral Nervous System

The peripheral nervous system can be divided into three working parts.

The autonomic nervous system (ANS) comprises the innervation of smooth muscle, cardiac muscle, and glands by sympathetic nerves (nerves issuing from the spinal cord to the chest region) and parasympathetic nerves (nerves issuing from the cranial and sacral regions of the spine). The two sets of nerves balance each other in that the sympathetic nerves prepare us for action in the face of danger (fight-or-flight response), while the parasympathetic nerves act to redress balance once the crisis has passed, slowing the breath, relaxing muscles, and lowering heart rate. The ANS has an involuntary unconscious response.

The somatic nervous system relates to the innervation of the skeleton or skeletal muscle, and has a voluntary or conscious response. It consists of forty-three pairs of peripheral nerves, which emerge from the CNS and link up the outer reaches of our anatomy. Each set consists of an afferent nerve conducting information from the peripheral body to the brain, and an efferent nerve, which transmits information from the brain to the body.

The enteric nervous system (mentioned in chapter one) can be classed separately because it is specific to the intestines and can operate independently from the CNS.

The Central Nervous System

The brain and spinal cord are the processing centers for information exchange. The brain is the major organ of the nervous system, for thought, speech, emotion and subtle control of bodily function. Chemicals produced in the brain affect the nerves themselves but also can directly affect cells via the blood stream and hormonal signals. The three main structures of the brain are the brain stem, cerebellum, and cerebrum (see diagram 5, page 176). Extending from the base of our brain are twelve pairs of cranial nerves, which innervate the muscles and sensory structures of the head and neck, except for the vagus nerve, which penetrates the abdominal cavity.

The brain stem and cerebellum are called "the animal brain," since they are the oldest evolutionarily and differ little from those of other mammals. The brain stem controls vital functions (breathing, blood pressure), and the cerebellum controls muscular coordination, balance, and posture. Both operate by reflex: a stimulus evokes an automatic response. Sensory information about temperature, pressure, and position is received from sensory receptors scattered throughout the body, after which our brain stem and cerebellum transmit what is perceived as the most appropriate response.

The forebrain consists of a central group of structures and nerve cell groups on top of the brain stem, and enclosing these is the relatively huge cerebrum. The right and left hemispheres of the cerebrum constitute nearly 70 percent of the weight of the entire nervous system!

The surface of the cerebrum is divided into distinct lobes — occipital, parietal, temporal and frontal — named after the main bones of the skull that overlie them. The outer surface of the cerebrum, or cerebral cortex, consists of "gray matter" in which nerve cells are arranged in six layers. This is considered the region of conscious thought, movement, and sensation.

Beneath the cerebral cortex, much of the cerebrum consists of tracts of nerve fibers forming "white matter." These tracts connect various areas of the cortex to each other and to nerve centers in the forebrain and brain stem. The entire brain and spinal cord is encased in three layers of membranes called meninges.

The cerebrospinal fluid, which circulates between two of these layers and within brain cavities, helps nourish the brain and cushion it from trauma. The brain as a whole has an extensive blood supply, which comes up through the carotid arteries running along each side of the front of the neck, and the two vertebral arteries that run parallel to the spinal cord.

As top priority to the nervous system, our brain receives about 20 percent of the cardiac output of blood with every heartbeat, and as much as 80 percent of the body's total blood circulation at any one time. Impaired blood and oxygen supply are the primary causes of brain dysfunction, as brain cells can survive only a few minutes without oxygen. Both blood and water carried in cerebrospinal fluid serve to deliver oxygen to the brain. Poor circulation and lack of oxygenation of the blood from shallow breathing will starve the brain, causing confusion, forgetfulness, and drowsiness. Most of us can remember a time in school when we experienced these symptoms, sitting for long periods with shallow breathing! Lack of fluid oxygen through lack of water intake can result in dehydration, which tightens the meninges and leads to headaches, lack of coordination, and heaviness of the head. Most herbs and foods that nourish the nervous system and brain also oxygenate it and improve overall circulation.

Herbs for the Nervous System

There are three groups of herbs for nervous disorders: *stimulants*, *relaxants*, and *restoratives*.

Herbal stimulants activate nerve tissue directly and are invaluable for illnesses of neurological breakdown, such as multiple sclerosis and muscular dystrophy. Herbs that contain some form of caffeine include coffee (too often overused in daily life), black and green teas, cola nut, yerba maté and guarana (*Paullinia cupana var. sorbilis*), which contains three times more caffeine than coffee by weight. Caffeine stimulates the adrenal glands, temporarily increasing circulation and body heat, reduces nausea, and in the correct dosage can relieve some headaches and help the brain focus; however, there are other stimulating herbs with similar effects that do not contain caffeine.

It's more often appropriate to stimulate our body's innate vitality with herbs that are pungent (spicy) and bitter tasting. They energize circulation primarily due to their high content of essential oil. These include cayenne pepper, ginger, garlic, peppercorn, mustard, horseradish, angelica, prickly ash bark, peppermint, cinnamon, camphor, bayberry, rosemary, juniper, sassafras, meadowsweet, clove, nutmeg, and cardamom. Note that many of these herbs act as digestive stimulants, dispersing blood by activating the heart and liver.

Today, stimulants are overused and thus have lost much of their medicinal efficacy. Constant firing of the nervous system doesn't allow for the replenishment of neurotransmitters or the parasympathetic nervous system. This wears on the nerves, slowing response time until they're no longer able to respond adequately. This can in turn desensitize or deplete other organs, resulting in such dangerous conditions as anxiety and adrenal failure.

Many herbs and foods (such as valerian and wine) can be stimulating in small doses yet depressing in larger ones. Dosage or tolerance for any herb is specific for each individual and may change depending on where you are in your life cycle, general health, and what's going on in your life. Stimulating herbs should not be used in cases of fluid depletion, hemorrhage, high blood pressure, and signs of overheating or inflammation — do not use stimulants in excessive amounts or continuously for long periods.

Herbal relaxants work by exercising an antispasmodic effect on peripheral nerves and muscles, or by soothing and protecting inflamed and irritated tissue. Sedative herbs — which include the power of flowers! — typically depress nervous and cardiac hyper-functioning, calm the mind, and promote rest. Hops flower, passion flower, chamomile, linden or lime blossom, lavender, California poppy, bitter orange flower / neroli, and rose are relaxants. Other calming herbs are lemon balm, motherwort, skullcap, valerian, wild lettuce, and St. John's wort. Herbs such as black cohosh, wild yam, lobelia, cramp bark, skunk cabbage root, black haw, kava, and valerian are powerful antispasmodics. Bitter and cooling herbs that treat irritability and inflammatory conditions (meningitis, encephalitis, rheumatic fever, heart palpitations) are European mistletoe (*Viscum album*), hawthorn, cactus grandiflorus, bean pod (*Phaseolus vulgaris*), passionflower, and dried or tinctured pasque flower. Demulcent herbs such as marshmallow, flax, aloe, slippery elm, and comfrey also help soothe and heal irritated nerve tissue.

Nervous system restoratives are herbs that repair, tone, and nourish nerve cells. A common misconception is that nerve damage can't be repaired; restorative herbs, however, along with essential fatty acids, can help the body repair the myelin sheath protecting nerve cells; and, with the help of circulatory stimulants, nerve tonics can aid in rebuilding, rerouting, and reconnecting nerve tissue. Herbs that work specifically on the spinal cord include gotu-kola, skullcap, basil, hyssop, blue cohosh, blue vervain, rosemary, oregano, and wild oats. Other herbs that build and strengthen nerves are clary sage, damiana, American and Asian ginsengs, ashwaganda, schizandra berry, cardamom, celery seed, eleuthero, jasmine flower, boneset, lemon peel, sesame seed, prickly ash bark, gingko, nettle, and all mints. Many of these are also adaptogenic, helping the body adapt to change and stress.

Nerve strength and repair also require particular nutrients from food, namely vitamins B_1, B_2, B_6, B_{12}, folic acid, and vitamin D, plus minerals — calcium, magnesium, potassium, phosphorus, and chloride. Other requirements are nutritional essential fatty acids and lecithin, *water* and *rest!* Spirulina and other super-greens, along with brewer's yeast, are among the highest-quality nerve foods there are, due to their high B vitamin content. Whole grains, celery, zucchini, pumpkin and its seeds, avocado, lettuce, broccoli, cauliflower, carrots, almonds, sesame seeds, pecans, and walnuts are all excellent nerve foods. High-protein foods such as bee pollen, soft-cooked eggs, and fish are also helpful.

Care of the Brain Under Stress

The brain uses glucose as a fuel. In fact, the brain uses 25 percent of the total energy the body produces. A steady supply of glucose for the brain is best achieved with a diet rich in complex carbohydrates and at least thirty grams of fiber a day. Fiber slows, and therefore steadies, the release of carbohydrates into the bloodstream. A diet rich in organic fresh fruits and vegetables provides the antioxidants our brain needs, since the fatty tissues of the brain are subject to oxidation. Chemicals in our foods, such as pesticides, artificial flavors and colors, plastic polymers, and heavy metals, along with chemicals found in animal tissues, nuts, and seeds, attach themselves to fats and act as nerve poisons, killing brain cells. Omega-3 fatty acids are also essential to the brain; a daily intake of these healthy oils equal to 15 – 20 percent of daily total calorie intake helps in membrane maintenance.

Chronic stress also kills brain cells by causing continual release of cortisol from the adrenal glands. Cortisol elevation is a common response to a stressful event, but when the event is over, cortisol levels return to normal. In the presence of long-term stress, cortisol levels remain high. Cortisol prevents the uptake of glucose by the part of our brain that helps sort and store memories. The halt of glucose uptake slows nerve-impulse transmission, resulting in cell death, which appears as memory loss. Certain anti-inflammatory drugs and steroids act on the brain in a similar manner. DHEA (dehydroepiandrosterone) is a precursor molecule to the synthesis of more than fifty hormones in the human body! In blood tests, it is common with people under constant stress to show high cortisol levels, but low DHEA levels, as the DHEA supplies in the adrenal glands are used to produce cortisol. Stress management is essential to care and repair of the brain and nervous system! Meditation and other relaxation techniques are among the most effective ways to lower cortisol levels and raise DHEA. Physical exercise and massage therapy also lower cortisol levels, while increasing blood supply to the brain, bringing fresh oxygen and nutrients to nourish brain cells. Mental exercise stimulates new connections between brain cells and helps restore memory, as do the herbs in the following formula:

Brain-booster Tea

3 parts each: gingko, gotu-kola, and peppermint

2 parts each: oatstraw, nettle, rosemary, rosehip, and hyssop

1 part each: basil, anise, nutmeg, stevia, and orange and lemon peels

Make a large pot and drink throughout the day!

The brain also requires large volumes of nutrient- and oxygen-rich blood; therefore, your brain is as clear as your blood is clean! Renewing the blood via bowel, liver, kidney, and lymph cleansing reduces the buildup of toxic residues, which can cause illnesses ranging from headache to dementia. Mostly water, the fluid surrounding the brain serves as a moat to protect and oxygenate neural tissue. If this moat begins to dry up, tissues dehydrate and long-term low oxygen levels leave neural tissue starved and under-functioning. If the moat becomes stagnant due to a combination of low water flow and poor circulation, heavy metals and other toxic debris accumulate. Stagnant water can no more nourish the brain than a stagnant pool can sustain fish. Substances like alcohol move quickly into the bloodstream and affect this protective moat by pulling oxygen off water molecules, consequently oxidizing brain tissue.

Drinking plenty of fresh, clean water and keeping your blood circulating are the simplest yet most effective ways to clear thinking!

All cells have a protective fatty-acid membrane called a phospholipid bilayer, and brain cells have especially thick ones. The membranes of brain cells are selective as to what passes through to the cell and what does not. Phosphatidylserine (PS), the primary food for this selective membrane that maintains cell integrity, is abundant in the membranes of brain cells and is important for allowing nutrients to enter the cells and wastes to leave. PS also helps brain cells conduct impulses and release adequate amounts of neurotransmitters.

Toxins that the liver is unable to process or eliminate are carried to our bloodstream and deposited in fatty tissues. Toxins are temporarily "safe" when tucked away in fatty tissues, but as we burn fat, they are released, accounting for "detox reactions" such as headaches.

From use and abuse and with aging, brain tissue begins to oxidize. Not age per se, the culprit is reduced circulation combined with toxins accumulated over a lifetime. Foods and herbs that are antioxidant to tissues are of great importance — and don't forget to *breathe deeply!*

Help For Common Ailments

Alzheimer's Disease

Alzheimer's disease and memory loss have been attributed to oxidation of brain cells from exposure to oxygen-robbing molecules such as pollutants, heavy metals, food additives, artificial sweeteners, alcohol, and drugs. Current research links memory loss with an overactive (overly stressed, overly defensive) immune system. Imbalance in immunity causes inflammation of the central nervous system and destruction of neurons transmitting and receiving signals to and from the brain. Anti-inflammatory herbs such as turmeric, green tea, ginger, holy basil, evening primrose oil, celery seed, bilberry (wild blueberry), feverfew, chrysanthemum, neem leaf, gentian, calendula, licorice, meadowsweet, myrrh, sage, wheatgrass, white poplar bark, willow bark, and wormwood are good allies. It helps to stop exposure to oxidants, and eliminate foods, beverages, and behaviors that provoke inflammatory reaction in the body. To activate brain cells, take this tincture daily:

Bouncy Brain Tincture

2 parts each: gingko, gotu-kola, and eleuthero

1 part each: hawthorn berry, rosemary, cayenne, licorice, and skullcap

½ part each: green tea and lemon peel

Add 2 drops of pure grapefruit essential oil per ounce of tincture.

Take 30 drops 3 to 4 times a day in hot water; let sit to dissipate alcohol first.

Eat antioxidant-rich foods, especially brightly colored fruits and vegetables, plus those high in vitamin E and omega-3 oils. Fresh vegetable juices and super-greens like wheatgrass, barleygrass, oatgrass, spirulina, and seaweeds deliver easily assimilated high-quality nutrients. Re-oxygenate the body by drinking plenty of purified water, breathing fresh air while exercising in nature, and using circulatory stimulants such as cayenne, gingko, gotu-kola, clove, ginger, garlic, and prickly ash bark. Finally, nothing is quite so clearing to the mind as cleansing and building the blood that feeds it. Toxins festering in the bowel continuously leak into the bloodstream and go to the head! Cleanse the bowel using gravity-fed high colonics, then flush the liver, and enjoy sharpened senses and sensibility.

Anxiety

Most of us have at some time experienced short-term anxiety in response to a situation. Anxiety or "fear spread thin" can become habitual and may arise out of over-stimulation of the sympathetic nervous system. Sensitive people and regular drug users are more prone to anxiety and chemical or hormonal imbalance. Anxiety can also occur during periods of great adrenal flux, for example during menopause or stressful situations. This is not an inherited condition. If you know you're more sensitive to the stimuli that cause fight-

or-flight response, it's important to be aware of what you allow yourself to be exposed to. Nurture yourself by creating a harmonizing environment in any way possible. Censor incoming stimuli (news, TV, radio, violent people, grating noise, electrical exposure) and take time each day to strengthen yourself by connecting with your center, lower belly, or hara (chi gong is excellent for this). Keeping the electromagnetic field of your body intact is also important, and this is where flower remedies, creative visualization, energy medicine, and shamanic healing are appropriate. Often in cases of chronic anxiety, there may be an underlying story or event that needs to be processed and released in some way.

Herbs that relax and restore will nourish the parasympathetic system, which quiets the sympathetic nervous system. Correct dosages of kava, valerian, and St. John's wort can be very helpful for three months. Over a longer period of time, a slight dependency can develop, necessitating steady decreases as you work on underlying issues, before stopping treatment altogether. Blue vervain, wild oats, lavender, linden or lime blossom, skullcap, lady's slipper root (*Cypripedium calceolus*), chamomile, lemon balm, damiana, seaweed, and California poppy can all be taken steadily for longer periods. Address any food allergies, cleanse all systems, consume foods that tone the nervous system, and stay away from stimulants and strong depressants. Essential oils of bergamot, tangerine, lavender, clary sage, melissa, linden, marjoram, ylang ylang, and rose can be of huge benefit, because scents go straight to the brain stem — the root of subconscious experience.

Concussion

Concussion is bruising of the brain caused by a blow to the head. Even minor concussions can have serious consequences if not cared for. Deal with the trauma immediately by first applying ice packs, taking homeopathic arnica and emergency tincture, and resting with both head and legs slightly elevated. Once initial shock has passed and any other wounds have been treated, get professional treatment in the form of cranial-sacral therapy, chiropractic care, acupressure, acupuncture, or reiki, and see a neurologist if necessary. For a week afterward, drink extra water with electrolytes, add Bach flower rescue remedy, and take antioxidants such as vitamins E and C. Eat antioxidant-rich foods, including plenty of super-greens, and use relaxing nervines and essential oils along with herbs that stimulate circulation. Take the time to recover and process the trauma emotionally.

Depression

Depression is a natural emotional response to bereavement, shock, or stressful life changes that force us to let go of the familiar. Short periods of depression are part of the need to go within and process change — it's usually unsettling, but if honored, this "fallow" period will soon give rise to new life. This is actually one of the best opportunities to cleanse the bowel, as it symbolically reinforces "letting go." Herbs that strengthen and support the process are wood betony (*Betonica officinalis*), cayenne, nutmeg, rosemary, lemon balm, damiana, blue vervain, skullcap, hawthorn berry, oatstraw, all ginsengs, borage flower and oil, St. John's wort, flaxseed oil, cola nut, basil, gingko, gotu-kola, cilantro, and calendula flower. Nearly all liver herbs help move depressed or stagnant energy. Anger is often below the surface of depression, so use liver cleansing as a tool to access and release deep feelings. Once again, essential oils prove invaluable: try basil, bergamot, lemon, orange, lavender, rose and jasmine. Flower remedies of particular help are gorse, monkey flower, tangerine, red sage, daffodil, and zinnia. For depression brought on by shifting hormones, please refer to chapter seven.

Chronic depression is not a normal state; it can be associated with micronutrient deficiency, hypothyroidism or other hormonal imbalances, unresolved anger or life trauma, abnormal metabolism of folic acid, vitamins B1 and B12, and deficiencies in vitamin D, calcium, and magnesium. Depression also correlates with low levels of eicosapentaneoic acid (EPA omega-3 fatty acid) in the blood, or a reduction of serotonin, an important neurotransmitter primarily found in the brain and large intestine. SAM-e can help by increasing levels of the neurotransmitters dopamine and serotonin. Foods high in the amino acid tryptophan, such as organic turkey and soy beans, will help in the formation of 5-HTP (5-hydroxytryptophan), which the body needs to produce serotonin. Deep-seated depression is a more complex issue, requiring an honest look at one's life, and the assistance of an experienced healthcare professional.

Insomnia

Occasional insomnia is a natural condition when triggered by a waxing-to-full moon, digesting a heavy meal late at night, or experiencing short-term stress. Chronic insomnia, however, can be the result of hormone imbalance, adrenal exhaustion, hyperactive thyroid, perpetual low-grade stress at work or at home, or disrupted sleep pattern due to nursing a newborn child, traversing time zones in travel, working a graveyard shift, or experiencing physical pain. Make note of the patterns of your insomnia, such as waking up between the same hours every night, and the days of the week or month as they correspond to activities or hormonal cycles.

Begin by honoring nature's cycles of natural light. The hormone melatonin, produced by the pineal gland, is a precursor to serotonin, and is regulated by Circadian rhythms (the twenty-four-hour solar / lunar cycle). Melatonin is produced in darkness while we sleep and is rapidly taken up by all tissues. Studies have shown that daily meditation can increase melatonin levels. Intense artificial light can disrupt physiological response to Circadian rhythm, so dim the lights or use candlelight before bed, and darken your bedroom at night if it is exposed to streetlights. Try to wake up with natural daylight when possible, and leave a window open to allow the sounds of nature yawning and stretching to welcome you to wakefulness. Winding down before bed means freeing yourself from electrical equipment — computer, video, TV — at least half an hour before sleeping. Listen to music, dance, read something inspirational, take a footbath or give yourself a foot massage, do some relaxed stretching and breathing exercises, or cuddle with someone you love. Sipping a cup of herbal tea an hour before bed can help lull you into dreamland.

Evening Peace Tea

3 parts chamomile

2 parts each: passion flower, valerian, and skullcap

1 part each: poppy flower, lavender flower, lemon balm, and spearmint

½ part stevia leaf or licorice root

¼ part lobelia

Steep, covered, 10 minutes, then add honey if desired.
Sip 1 to 2 cups an hour or two before bed.

This formula also works as a tincture and can be kept by the bedside and taken as needed.

Migraines

Migraines occur when arteries in the brain constrict and then become swollen with fluid, creating major pressure on the brain. This can result from hormonal shifts, sudden changes in barometric pressure, high altitude, allergies, stress, constipation, overwork, eyestrain, or neck tension. Place an ice pack at the back of your neck, touching the base of your skull. Lie down like this for immediate relief from a headache and to reduce the severity of a migraine. Headaches occur with higher frequency in people who are high achievers (whether outwardly or inwardly). Chewing on a bit of fresh feverfew each day can help prevent or minimize migraines. Taking a tincture or capsules of feverfew six days a week for three months can also reduce their occurrence.

Other helpful herbs are rosemary, blue vervain, and butterbur rhizome or leaves (*Petasites hybridensis*), which decreases inflammation and spasms in blood-vessel walls. Avoid foods that aggravate migraines: coffee, black tea, cocoa, chocolate, yeast extract, oranges, bananas, potatoes, hard cheeses, moldy cheese (essentially all cheese), alcohol, cream, and pickles. Rest, acupressure, deep breathing, and sleep are often the final relief, especially since we do our deepest breathing when we sleep. Essential oils of lavender, rosemary, and peppermint should be used immediately upon onset of pain.

Use them topically by dabbing on your temples, the nape of your neck, and your belly and feet, or use in a diffuser. Try sipping the following tea, before symptoms become severe:

 ## Headache-free Tea

2 parts each: wood betony and skullcap

1 part each: chamomile and meadowsweet flower

½ part each: hops and peppermint

Steep, covered, for 10 to 15 minutes.

Note that hedge nettle herb (Stachys palustris) has a similar action and can be substituted for wood betony. Drink this tea as a preventative or at onset of headache.

Neurological Pain

Neurological pain, or neuralgia, whatever the cause, can be unbearable. Herbs for pain are most effective when taken internally *and* applied topically as compresses or salves to the site of pain. Neuralgia from shingles (herpes zoster) can be treated with hops, Jamaican dogwood (*Piscidia piscipula*), lobelia, motherwort, rue, skullcap, pasque flower, clove, celery seed, and St. John's wort herb as well as homeopathic St. John's wort or homeopathic *gelsenium*. Neuralgia from skeletal nerve compression (sciatica) is eased by compresses of a combination of arnica, ginger, and hops, plus application of essential oils such as marjoram, wintergreen, cayenne, mustard, birch, camphor, oregano, and basil. Antispasmodic herbs — Jamaican dogwood, wild yam, black cohosh, kava, skunk cabbage root and skullcap — work well with anti-inflammatory herbs. Valerian, hops, blue vervain, and California poppy root are nearly always appropriate for nerve pain.

Persistent intensive pain in any part of the body is debilitating to the entire nervous system. Pain is often the cause of insomnia, leading to steady wear and tear on the body, and giving rise to anxiety, heart palpitations, digestive upset, and depression. Pain management must be approached from a multitude of angles; professional help can be of great value. Acupuncture, acupressure, therapeutic massage, and energy work such as reiki are all excellent adjunct therapies.

Beyond the Brain

Our brain is so much more than its physiology. The right and left hemispheres are engaged in a constant dance, taking turns at leading and following, depending on the music of our moods and sensory input. A variety of stimuli in daily life present the brain with delightful challenges as well as serious stress. Sometimes our perception of stress locks our brains into over-activity on one side, to the detriment of the other, causing brain imbalance.

Brain imbalance can result from physical stress (due to injury, spinal problems, chemical exposure, or drugs), mental stress, or emotional causes. Brain imbalance is subtle, but can show itself in "spacey" behavior, momentary confusion or blanking out, slurred or stuttering speech, inability to deal with small things, sudden postural changes, loss of balance, or sudden change in visual acuity. In any case, we are no longer operating at our full potential. Various therapies rebalance the brain by reconnecting the hemispheres of our brain and then reconnecting our brain with the rest of our body! Feldenkreis therapy, alphabiotics, brain gym, yoga, certain forms of meditation, music therapy, cranial-sacral therapy, somatic release techniques, Bowen technique, and polarity can all help achieve this end. Take time to explore this vast frontier we call the mind — and the brain that houses it.

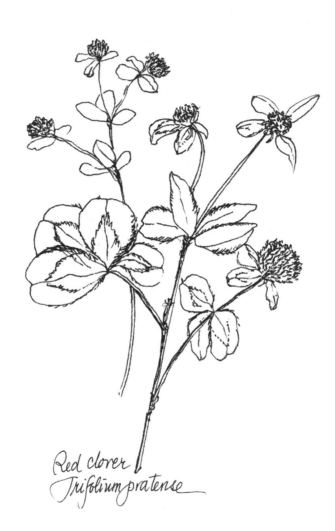

Red clover
Trifolium pratense

Chapter Nine

Lymph System:
Lymph Vessels and Tools for Activating Lymph

When we try to pick out anything by itself,
We find it hitched to everything else in the universe.

John Muir

If you imagine the bloodstream as mirroring the earth's primary waterways, the lymph system symbolizes secondary tributaries and the natural drainage system that occurs both above and below ground. Every moment trillions of water molecules in the soil merge with one another as they wend their way to lakes and oceans, in the same way that fluid between our cells, interstitial fluid, is ever migrating back to the largest lymph vessels of our thoracic cavity. This constant recycling and renewing of fluid happens from the most macroscopic level to the most microscopic level, every moment of every day, whether we notice it or not. In fact, we rarely are aware of it until the flow comes to a halt — whether a stream becomes blocked with silt, or our tissues become uncomfortably swollen. What exactly is this invisible movement of fluid?

Galium aparine
Cleavers

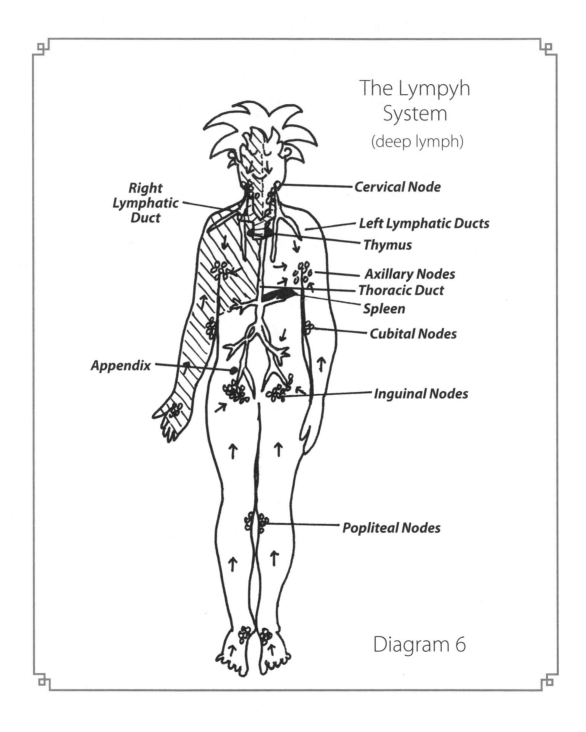

The Lympyh
System
(deep lymph)

Right
Lymphatic
Duct

Cervical Node

Left Lymphatic Ducts

Thymus

Axillary Nodes

Thoracic Duct

Spleen

Cubital Nodes

Appendix

Inguinal Nodes

Popliteal Nodes

Diagram 6

The lymphatic system is a network of highly permeable lymph capillaries that are closely associated with veins throughout most of our body. They assist veins by collecting excess fluids from within body tissues and returning those fluids to the heart. Lymph fluid is composed of waste materials, proteins, fats (extracted from capillary beds), interstitial fluid, white blood cells, salts, and water. The system is passive system, in that transport of this fluid through the lymph vessels depends upon external pressure or friction (muscle contraction or manual manipulation), blood circulation, overall tissue pressure, and body heat. This differs from our blood, which is actively pumped with each heartbeat. One-way valves in the lymphatic system ensure that whatever moves in always flows forward, moving toward the center of the body. There are two types of lymph vessels: the superficial vessels and the deep lymph vessels (see diagram 6, page 194).

The superficial lymph consists of vessels just beneath the skin and surrounding all organs, the lymph flowing through vessels of progressively larger diameter up the legs, arms, and torso, and down the neck and upper chest. The right side (arm, chest, neck, head, top curvature of the liver, and right side of the heart) drains into its own lymph duct, the right lymphatic duct. Lymph vessels of the left side of the body and lower extremities, liver, spleen — and substances absorbed from the gastrointestinal tract (principally fats) — drain into the left lymphatic duct, then both ducts drain into the largest lymph vessel, the thoracic duct. These ducts are part of the deep lymph, which pours approximately one and a half quarts (1.15 liters) of fluid back into the heart every twenty-four hours.

The protein that the lymphatic system returns to the bloodstream represents about one-fourth to one-half of all circulating plasma proteins. Lymphatic return is the only means by which proteins that enter the tissues can return to the blood. If protein is not returned from the tissues, it accumulates there and draws fluid (mostly water) from the blood capillaries into body tissues, producing severe edema and swelling (due to excessive water retention). This dehydration of the bloodstream promotes hardening of the arteries and thickening of the blood.

Situated along the course of main lymphatic vessels are the lymph nodes — small filtering stations shaped like kidney beans and ranging in size from a coriander seed to that of an almond. These serve to filter off particulate matter (i.e., bacteria) and are the major sites of lymphocyte (white blood cell) production. Lymph nodes are gathered in fairly well defined groups along the sides and back of our neck, in our armpits, groin, and at the root of our lungs near the large veins of the abdomen and pelvis. Tissue similar to lymph tissue is found in the spleen, tonsils, adenoids, and along the digestive tract. Only cartilage, bone, epithelium, and tissues of the central nervous system are devoid of lymphatic vessels.

Loving Your Lymph

To reduce the burden on your lymph system, it's imperative to severely limit or exclude the ingestion of animal products (which are high in saturated fats and pathogenic organisms) and eat only organically grown produce, legumes, and whole grains when possible. Any additives, preservatives, colorings, flavorings, alcohol, or foods high in theobromine (such as coffee or chocolate), plus other poisons should be avoided. Consumption of dairy products, fried foods, and wheat-gluten products congests our lymphatic system considerably.

Foods that assist lymphatic flow by increasing capillary filtration rate are raw chilies, ginger, garlic, uncooked black pepper, mustard, horseradish, cinnamon, clove, allspice, basil, bay, cardamom, coriander, cumin, oregano, eucalyptus, peppermint, rosemary, thyme, kelp, lemon, purslane, and cider vinegar. These pungent flavors contain aromatic oils, which stimulate all organs while reducing the growth of microbes in the body. For those who lose weight easily, combine pungent flavors with neutral and sweet flavors (i.e., squash and yams) to keep metabolism balanced. Note that an excess of sugary foods and drinks — even natural ones — can cause swelling of the lymph glands and lowered immunity. Most important, drink plenty of filtered water!

The lymphatic system depends upon all eliminative channels (skin, lungs, kidneys, tear ducts, ears and bowels) to carry accumulated waste out of the body so that it can continue processing incoming material. Clearing and toning lymph vessels includes cleansing and opening ALL eliminative channels. The bowels are a good place to start, since deep lymph vessels run just behind them.

Lymph-lovin' Tea

1 part each: mullein leaf and flower, red clover blossom, blue violet, peppermint, and calendula

¼ part lobelia

Steep for 15 – 30 minutes, strain, and drink throughout the day between meals.

Primary Lymph Herbs

Since the lymphatic system is actually a part of the circulatory system, any blood-cleansing herbs, or alteratives, are effective in cleansing and supporting our lymph tissues. Herbs with anti-microbial action, such as garlic and cloves, also serve to cleanse or disinfect lymphatic fluids. Diaphoretics are heat-producing herbs, which assist when infection is present by raising body temperature, thereby increasing the flow of lymph fluid and effectively stimulating immune response. Diuretic herbs stimulate kidney function, hepatics stimulate liver function, and both promote cleansing of the lymphatic system. Note that many of the herbs listed below are also immune- and skin-supporting herbs! These brief descriptions do not account for other healing effects they have on the body.

Herbs Particularly Supportive to the Lymphatic System

Burdock Root (*Arctium lappa*) is excellent for relieving lymphatic congestion and helps remove excess fat from the tissues. It strengthens and tones as it cleanses the bloodstream, and is specifically used to treat swellings, blood poisoning, arthritis, rheumatism, and cancer.

Blue Flag (*Iris versicolor*) is good for dissolving accumulations, especially where liver congestion and spleen enlargement are involved. Blue flag addresses general disharmony due to high toxin levels, as well as skin complaints. Its dissolving nature helps clear stones from the bladder, liver, and gallbladder.

Calendula Flower (*Calendula officinalis*) is excellent for removing lymph congestion by reducing lipids (fats) held in the lymph. A gentle capillary stimulant, it softens and dissolves lipids, and has an astringent effect on tissues, while reducing venous blood stagnation. Its antimicrobial action is effective in treating herpes, staphylococcus, and thrush.

Chaparral Leaf (*Larrea tridentata, L. californica, L. divaricala*). The resinous leaves and stems of this bush are a potent healer, and are used specifically for treating cancer, eczema, tumors, and arthritis. Chaparral oxygenates interstitial fluids, and its bitter, pungent flavor moves deep lymph, especially of the liver; it should not be used for more than three weeks at a time, and is contraindicated in cases of spleen deficiency.

Cleavers (*Galium aparine*) is used in treating enlarged lymph nodes (tonsils, and adenoids, etc.), skin diseases and eruptions, along with ulcers and tumors that are a result of poor lymphatic drainage. Cleavers is a nutrient-packed herb that tones the waters and dissolves excess fats of the body. Make a plant juice by placing cleavers and spring water in the blender to create a green drink — using the freshly picked herb is most effective.

Echinacea (*Echinacea angustifolia, E. purpurea, E. pallida*). Use the root, leaf, flower, or seed of this herb to assist the body in ridding itself of microbial infections. Its action increases T-cell transformation, interferon production, and the stimulation of lymphocytes, leukocytes, and macrophage activity (the lymphatic cleanup crew). Echinacea reduces mucus over-secretion by stimulating capillary circulation, and is both heat-clearing, and dissolving, thus useful for inflammations, blood poisoning, and swollen glands.

Figwort (*Scrophularia nodosa, S. marilandica*) leaf and flower are cooling and drying, thus helpful in decongesting impacted lymph tissue and dissolving hardened interstitial tissue nodules called *scrofula*. It's especially helpful for stagnant lymph in the liver, bowels, skin, and pancreas.

Jasmine Flower (*Jasminum grandiflorum*) has long been used in India for the treatment of cancerous lymph nodes, tumors, and viral infections. Its flower is considered cooling, calming, and strengthening to the lymphatic system. This is also true of jasmine essential oil.

Mullein (*Verbascum thapsus*) leaves and flowers loosen mucus throughout the entire lymphatic system, especially the respiratory parts. It also reduces pain and swelling of the lymph nodes, and can be used as an ear oil (to loosen lymph congestion in the ears) or externally as a poultice or fomentation for swollen glands or tumors. It can be taken daily to reduce mucus congestion.

Poke Root (*Phytolacca americana*) leaves and root are strong lymph cleansers, especially good for addressing painful, swollen, hard lymph glands, cysts, and cancerous tumors. It is best used simultaneously in external (poultices) and internal applications (in combination with other supportive herbs) for specific conditions. Do not use for more than two weeks at a time. The *fresh* raw root and berries are poisonous to eat.

Red Clover Flowers (*Trifolium pratense*) effectively thin the blood and promote expectoration of mucus from the body. Red clover assists the lymph system by removing obstructions in the vessels, particularly of the liver, skin, breast, reproductive organs, kidneys, and lungs. A nurturing, blood-thinning, restorative, and moistening herb, it has a mild yet deep-acting nature and with strong anti-cancer effects.

Red Root (*Ceanothus americanus*). The root of this herb is decongesting for lymph and stimulating to the spleen (dispelling damp heat and relieving spleen enlargement). It works aggressively with the lymph system in addressing swollen glands as well as non-fibrous ovarian cysts and cancerous conditions. For a milder, toning action, the leaves can be taken as tea.

Many herbs help cleanse and decongest lymph by supporting the blood stream, lungs, liver, or kidneys, including dandelion, wild cherry bark, clove, sarsaparilla, American ephedra, goldenseal, Oregon grape, sage, walnut leaf, pau d'arco bark, and yellow dock. Asian herbs to treat the lymph system include forsythia (*Forsythia suspensa*) or "Lian qiao," honeysuckle (*Lonicera japonica*) or "Jin Yin Hua," and pinella (*Pinella ternate*) or "Ban Xia."

Naturally, a healthy lymphatic system is contingent upon a healthy body! The herbs mentioned can be taken internally as infusions, tinctures, or capsules, or externally as poultices and fomentations. It's always best to begin with small amounts of one or two herbs taken consistently over a two- to three-week period, to assess how your body responds and whether an herb is the right match for you. Even without the use of particular herbs, you can cleanse the lymphatic system by flushing it with liquids for three days.

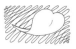 ### The Three-day Lymphatic Flush

This cleanse is incredibly effective if you've been following the Revitalizing Diet and have experienced a thorough bowel cleanse within the past month. To move excess mucus from the intestines, add this flush to the end of your bowel cleanse.

Three days is considered the minimum time it takes to flush out lymph vessels and nodes throughout the body. For the week prior, stay on a vegan (no animal products), flourless, sugar-free, soy-free diet. One or two days before the flush, eat only raw fruit, seeds, nuts, sprouts, and vegetables. Choose *one* juice you wish to stay with for the full three days; apple, grape, or carrot are recommended for their alkalinizing effect. The only other juice you'll be drinking during the cleanse is prune juice. Liquids should be at room temperature or warmer.

Below is the protocol for each of the three days:

Upon rising drink one glass of water, followed by eight to ten ounces of prune juice with the juice of one lemon (to promote bowel movement). Sip this slowly ("chew" it so it mixes well with your saliva), then slowly drink alternate glasses of your chosen juice (fresh-pressed is best) and filtered water all day long until you have consumed as close to a gallon of juice and one gallon of water as possible. You may wish to add water and / or lemon juice to each glass of juice to reduce sweetness. In addition, mix together or take each separately 1 to 3 times a day:

1 tablespoon oil of wheat germ, flax, or borage

1 tablespoon apple cider vinegar

1 teaspoon kelp or dulse powder

¼ – 1 teaspoon cayenne pepper

1 tablespoon of organic blackstrap molasses can be taken if desired.

By the end of the day, you'll have consumed nearly two gallons of liquid, unless you weigh less than 125 lb. (57 kg), are of fragile health, or have compromised kidneys, in which case you drink less, as appropriate for your situation. Anti-microbial herbs such as garlic and echinacea may be taken during this time, as well as bowel-supporting herbs if necessary. Your bowel must be eliminating each day; if your bowel is sluggish, drink another glass of prune juice with lemon before bed.

During the three days, it's important to keep your lymph moving with one hour of modest exercise (thirty minutes of which should be aerobic or opening to the lungs). Brisk walking in fresh air is very effective, as are biking, swimming, dancing, and yoga. The emphasis is on deep breathing combined with stretching and movement of the muscular-skeletal system. Very rigorous and competitive sports are best avoided, since the body needs to channel energy into eliminating toxins. Other activities that augment the cleansing process are skin brushing, water therapy, bodywork, meditation, and *rest*. If you're feeling tired, *don't push it*! Ideally, the three-day cleanse is carried out when you have more personal time for yourself, because previously "stuck" emotions may also move out of the body. Consciously acknowledging and staying with this emotional energy will help release it. As toxins are released from the body, you may experience some unpleasant physical effects such as nausea, headache, backache, aching feet, or dizziness and disorientation — usually only on the first day. This is generally a sign of progress as toxins are released in your body to be eliminated.

By the second day these symptoms typically disappear and your energy will increase, although this varies from person to person. If, however, you're still experiencing the unpleasant effects of toxic clearing on the third day, then further bowel and liver cleansing are recommended. As with any cleanse, it's imperative that you listen to the wise inner voice of your body; if at any time you feel a cleanse is too much or too fast, then slow it down or stop altogether.

After the third day of lymph cleansing, the juice fast can be broken with raw fruits before noon — don't forget to take your time and chew your food well! Raw vegetables, salads, and vegetable juices can be taken from noon until four hours before bed. In the late evening, only fruit and fruit juices may be consumed. On the fourth day, begin again with fresh fruit and fruit juices until noon, and slowly introduce soft, cooked foods in the evening.

This flush should leave you feeling renewed and revitalized. Healthy adults can do this safely up to four times a year.

 ### *Alternative Three-day Lymph Flush*

This cleanse is labor intensive, but well worth it! It's a very effective flush, and more satisfying for those who become "tired of sweet" juice cleanses. As with any cleanse, it's extremely important to be sure your bowels are fully eliminating and all channels of elimination (skin, kidneys, lungs) are open, too. The schedule for each of the three days:

Upon rising: Drink a glass of spring or distilled water. Follow this by juicing one organic lemon including the rind (for this, Meyer lemons are best) with a 2-inch square of fresh ginger root. Add to this 8 ounces of warm water and 1 teaspoon of raw honey, and sip slowly.

Breakfast: Make a 12-ounce juice of 4 ounces celery, 3 ounces parsley, 2 ounces carrot, 2 ounces beet, and a thumb-sized piece of ginger root (garlic optional). Add another 6 ounces of water and drink it slowly, being sure to "chew" your juice (mix it well with your saliva) as you do.

Between meals: Drink plenty of spring or distilled water (*a gallon a day*) and herbal teas like Lymph-lovin' Tea, as desired.

Mid-morning: Drink 8 ounces of distilled / spring water with the juice of one whole organic lemon, a teaspoon of cayenne pepper, with maple syrup to taste.

Lunch: Prepare the following soup:

> *Steam a cup chopped string or green beans for 5 minutes, then add a cup chopped celery and continue steaming 5 more minutes; finally, add a cup chopped zucchini and steam another 5 minutes. Put all of the steamed vegetables in the blender with some Vital Broth (recipe below), and add 1 to 2 teaspoons of freshly chopped parsley. Season to taste with Bragg Liquid Aminos, onion, garlic, basil, thyme, turmeric, etc., and blend well. Sip it warm. Add 1 teaspoon of flax oil and 1 teaspoon of olive oil to the soup to activate the liver. Enjoy!*

Mid-afternoon: Drink 8 ounces of the same vegetable juice combo you had at breakfast.

One hour before dinner: Drink 8 ounces warm distilled / spring water with 1 tablespoon raw apple cider vinegar (add supertonic if desired).

Dinner: Relish a bowl of *Vital Broth:*

Use equal parts of thick potato peelings (using the entire potato is fine — use small ones), carrot tops, onions, garlic, celery tops (and / or whole celery), kelp, and any herbs as desired. This particular recipe doesn't use carrots, beets, or other greens so as to intentionally reduce certain acids in the body. Bring the crudely chopped ingredients to a boil in distilled or spring water, turn down to a simmer, and cook, covered, for 1 hour. Strain. Drink only the broth. It's helpful to do this in a pasta pot so you can just lift the vegetables right out of the broth. You can make a three-day batch and store the remaining broth in the refrigerator. It's fine to switch the lunch and dinner meals if you desire.

Two hours before bedtime: Drink 8 ounces of the same breakfast vegetable juice.

Once you complete this cleanse, slowly introduce raw foods and juices, then steamed vegetables and grains.

There is no "Help for Common Ailments" section in this chapter, as sluggish lymph flow manifests in a wide variety of ways: excess mucus, respiratory ailments, swollen glands, cellulite, water retention, a compromised immune system, allergies, and cancer — all of which are addressed in other chapters. Such manifestations are signs that blood and lymph need to be activated and excess toxins eliminated. Below are some wonderful tools for enhancing the action of the lymphatic system. These supporting and toning methods may be employed daily, weekly, or monthly as outlined below.

A Hot Bath

There's nothing quite like a hot bath for moving mucus in the body! For your lymphatic system to truly benefit, a hot bath should be taken on an empty stomach just before going to bed (you might wish to skip dinner). Drinking diaphoretic teas such as peppermint, ginger, and yarrow help turn up the internal body heat before and during the bath. Fill the tub with the hottest water comfortable, add one cup of Epsom salts and one cup of sea salt, plus any appropriate essential oil(s) or herbs, then *soak* — get red in the face and let your perspiration flow!

Try to stay in the bath for at least twenty minutes so you affect the deep lymph. This time, *do not* rinse with cold water to end (though you'll likely want to); simply get out and sit down on your towel on the rim of the tub (or stool) and let your skin continue to perspire while you slowly sip room-temperature lemon water. After three to five minutes, pat your skin dry, put on warm cotton pajamas (flannel is best) and go to bed.

Make sure you have plenty of drinking water at hand. Pile on the blankets to retain heat. You should be uncomfortably warm, but stay that way — the idea is to perspire much of the night. In the morning, take a tepid shower, change your bedding as needed, drink plenty of water, and eat lightly all day.

The basis of this treatment is to create a feverish state that causes the lymph fluid to race about, collecting excess mucus and raising antibody action. Toxins are released through the sebaceous glands in the skin. It's particularly helpful for clearing up low-grade infections shown by swollen glands, as for instance at the first sign of cold or flu. You'll likely wake up to drink water several times during the night as you lose fluid, but by morning you'll be feeling great! Rub essential oil of thyme or apply *garlic paste* to your feet before bed to increase immune defense.

Garlic Paste

Crush fresh cloves of garlic and mince into a paste. Apply to feet that have been thinly coated with non-petroleum jelly or an olive-oil-based ointment (to protect the skin on the soles of your feet). Cover each foot with a plastic bag or other nonabsorbent material and then a sock. The oil of garlic will saturate your body as you sleep, and drive away lingering viruses (and perhaps a few family members!).

Alternate Hot and Cold Showers

As a general rule, one should always end a hot shower with cool water to close the pores of the skin and reseal the body from outside influences. Our skin is the body's first defense mechanism, and the superficial lymph system lies just underneath, acting as the second line of defense. Hot water opens our pores and moves our blood, but this opening also allows the uptake of outside influences, such as bacteria, viruses, and climatic changes that may cause disturbance to the body. Closing the doors with cold water (however briefly) will help protect your body from illness. Alternating hot and cold water takes this even further by stimulating circulation, which in turn stimulates lymphatic fluids and your body overall (even the brain, and most certainly your voice). This is done in the shower by simply standing under hot water for several minutes and then turning the water to cold for as long as you can stand it, then going back to hot, and repeating these alterations up to seven times. Be gentle on yourself by gradually working up to longer periods of cold water. Always finish with cool water.

Hot and cold treatments can also be done by alternating a hot bath with a cold shower or plunge, or even alternating an ice pack with a hot water bottle. If you have a specific injury, say to knee or shoulder, you can treat that area this way, stimulating blood flow and oxygen to the tissues, thus speeding up the healing process. If you want to relax and revitalize the lower back and pelvic area, then take alternate hot and cold sitz baths. A sitz bath is simply a mini-bath in which you submerge only your lower torso to upper thighs. The smallest application of this method is to take alternate hot and cold footbaths, which can serve to stimulate all body functions. Hot and cold treatment is not recommended for those suffering persistent chilblains or weakened heart. At all times, use your own discretion as to how hot is "hot" and how cold is "cold." If you're vocalizing and breathing strongly, you probably have the temperature just right!

Aromatherapy

Molecules of plant oils can enter the olfactory system, going straight to the brain, or slip through the skin and enter the bloodstream where they have a powerful effect on the body. Even if our noses don't respond to the scent, the cells of our body do, so the healing potential of essential oils should never be underestimated. A great many oils are available, each with a slightly different effect on the body. You can consult aromatherapy books, but don't be afraid to experiment on your own. A good rule of thumb: *always smell oils before buying them.* If you enjoy the scent and it stimulates positive feelings, then it's worth the investment. Oil quality can vary considerably — be sure they're *pure* and preferably organic.

Oils that are beneficial to the lymphatic system include fennel, celery, grapefruit, cypress, and juniper, which have a strong diuretic action; while oregano, lemon, lemon grass, basil, rosemary, sage, and thyme all have a strong immune action. Please note that most of these oils are contraindicated in pregnancy. Drops of essential oil can be used in a bath, in an oil burner, in water as a body mist — use your imagination, but remember that a little goes a long way! If you want to use them directly on your skin, dilute them in a carrier oil such as almond, apricot kernel, or jojoba. A nice way to introduce yourself to the wonder of essential oils is to receive an aromatherapy massage.

Color and Sound Therapy

Working with color and sound is a wonderful way to enhance your energy and overall healing process. The body has seven primary chakras or gates of energy, which correspond to the endocrine glands. The first chakra, associated with the color red and the base of the spine, is linked with a small gland at the end of the tailbone. The second or sacral chakra is associated with the color orange and the reproductive glands. It also influences the lymphatic system, skin, reproductive organs, kidneys, bladder, and circulation. The third chakra is associated with the color yellow and is linked to the liver and pancreas. The fourth chakra is associated with the color green and the thymus gland; turquoise too is a color used to boost the immune system. Blue is the color associated with the fifth chakra and the thyroid, while indigo is linked with the sixth chakra — the third eye — and the pituitary gland. The seventh chakra, associated with bright white or sometimes soft violet, is found at the top of the head where the pineal gland is located. Working with color means more than just wearing it and having it around you. It requires visualizations in which you breathe in the color and imagine it flowing through your body. There are also sounds associated with each chakra, as well as musical tones for each color. Books and tapes are available to guide you in this direction.

Hydrotherapy

Water therapies are some of the oldest, time-proven methods of natural healing. Various spas and healing centers the world over offer treatments ranging from the well-known Turkish bath to being sprayed down with high-powered hoses. Described below are effective treatments easily carried out in your own home; providing you have hot and cold running water and a shower and / or bathtub (preferably both), you can create your own spa!

Lifestyle

If you have a healthy lifestyle, but your lymphatic system is still burdened or suffering, consider the environment you're living in. Illnesses that affect the blood and lymph are often caused by exposure to low levels of pollutants on a daily basis. Common causes for lymphatic congestion might be due to cigarette smoke, pesticide sprays, petroleum products, household cleaners, dust, molds, sulfites in foods or beverages, and chemicals in paints, printer inks, and plastics, etc. Electromagnetic radiation from cell phones, wireless phones, poorly wired buildings, microwaves, and cell towers all cause cellular miscommunication, thus havoc to your health. Start paying attention to the elements in your living and working environment in order to develop an awareness of how they affect your body. Make any changes necessary to eliminate things that disturb your equilibrium. Keep supporting your lymph system so it can handle environmental stress, but if your surroundings are literally making you sick, consider moving if you can. Make room for change, even in the most seemingly impossible circumstances.

Your environment may also be energetically or emotionally toxic. If you spend the majority of your time in places of geopathic stress, you might be suffering all kinds of odd symptoms caused by depletion or distortion of earth energies. If you suspect geopathic stress to be a factor, seek guidance from a skilled geomancer, *Feng Shui* master, or spiritual healer.

Emotional stress caused by constant output of negative energy by those around you can have the same harmful effects. In such cases one must confront the situation and seek a workable solution. You might also have to do more to fortify your personal boundaries. Use your intention to center your mind on life's essentials — love and joy.

Finally, semiannual to quarterly cleansing of the eliminatory systems of the body, specifically the bowel, liver, and kidneys, reduces load on the lymphatic system and toxin load to organs and fatty tissue in general. Schedule regular cleanses into your yearly calendar as a part of your own wellness program, and get emphatic about your lymphatics!

Manual Lymphatic Drainage Massage (MLD)

While nearly all forms of massage are beneficial to the lymphatic system, MLD is used specifically to stimulate circulation of the lymph fluids, with the pumping motion encouraging but not forcing the flow of lymph. MLD is helpful for excess fluid retention in general (edema) and your lymph vessels in particular. It's also an assisting treatment during cleansing, or helpful as a post-illness treatment. Receiving MLD post-operatively, or after radiation and chemotherapy, is important because body functions become "stunned" after such severe handling and there are copious amounts of toxic substances in the system. A series of treatments should be undergone over a three-week to three-month period, depending upon one's condition. It is also beneficial after any illness that has left the body weakened (see the resource list to find a certified practitioner near you).

Movement and Meditation

As mentioned previously, proper function of the lymphatic system depends on movement of the muscular-skeletal system. There's movement that involves greater cardiac output, such as water exercise and aerobic exercise, and there's movement involving deep stretching of the tissues. It's not enough to have one without the other — both types of movement are necessary, and any exercise program must include a balance between them. Exercise that increases cardiac output, speeds lymphatic flow, and opens elimination channels is detoxifying. Exercise that combines thorough stretching of connective tissue with deep breathing feeds oxygen to all cells of the body, balances the acid-base ratio, and has an antioxidant effect on the system.

Stretching and relaxing the mind, meditation is a form of movement — of the spirit. There are various forms of sitting and walking meditations, so experiment! Like all body systems, the lymph system is influenced by thoughts and feelings. The web of superficial lymph vessels essentially provides a protective watery membrane for our bodies, in the same way that amniotic fluid protects us in the womb. In both cases, these "water webs" transport nutrients and waste materials and protect us from infection. The webs provide a way of taking in or keeping out the energies around us, as part of the greater web of life. Find out how you process the energy of your surroundings and how you relate to your environment in general. Visualization techniques are a wonderful tool, and the best methods are often the ones you create for yourself.

Mud or Clay Wrap

This part of spa life can be done at home! You'll need about a pint of wet clay (white, red, or green) or good mud (moor, Red Sea, or dead sea) and an expendable bed sheet. Take a warm bath or shower while you soak the sheet in hot water. After bathing, pat yourself barely dry, then slather wet clay or mud (into which you can mix seaweed, herbs, essential oils, or flower essences) all over your body and face (it would help if you had a friend nearby to apply the clay to your back). Then thoroughly wring out the wet sheet, carefully wrap it around you, and lie down in a warm place wrapped up in plastic or a foil sheet covered with blankets for fifteen to twenty minutes, depending on the type of clay or mud you use. White clay is mild and can stay on for longer periods, but red and especially green clays are highly active and sometimes irritating, so may require less time. Unwrap and scrub off under a warm shower (do not use soap), end with cool water, and pat or air-dry your skin. Follow with a sesame-oil massage to nourish dry skin.

Salt Scrubs and Ice Rubs

Sound tempting? This is an ancient method of pulling toxins and excess fluid out of lymph vessels. Start by sitting naked on a stool in your empty bathtub, making sure the room is comfortably warm (better yet, do this outside if it's warm enough). Rinse your skin lightly with warm water and have with you a pint or half-liter mix of two-thirds fine crystal sea salt to one-third Epsom salts. Add a bit of essential oil such as rosemary and lemon if desired, along with some carrier oil (olive, sesame, almond), plus enough hot water to make the salt mix clump easily. Then take a handful of salt and rub it well into your skin, starting at the feet and working your way up in the same direction as with skin brushing. Do this thoroughly all over your body — ask someone to help you salt-scrub your back.

As the salt sticks, it pull toxins and excess fluids out of your body, so it's important to drink plenty of water for the rest of the day after the treatment. When you're finished applying the salt, rest five minutes before rinsing off thoroughly with tepid water.

An ice rub follows the same principle, except you rub crushed ice all over your body to stimulate the system by bringing circulation (thus heat) to the surface. The salt scrub is more eliminating and detoxifying, while the ice rub is more toning — both are invigorating!

Sauna

Saunas are stimulating and cleansing for the skin, lymph, and lungs — especially if you chant in the sauna. The true healing aspect is taking a *cold water* plunge or cold shower between sessions of dry heat. Three rounds of hot air / cold water are recommended — always ending with cold. Replace lost electrolytes with a tea made from nettle, raspberry, and rosehip, or with lemon water with raw honey, sea vegetables, or fresh-squeezed fruit or vegetable juices.

Skin brushing

This is a daily activity that bestows reverence on the superficial lymph vessels, and your skin will appreciate it, too! It takes only minutes, and can be done just before you bathe or shower. It requires a natural, firm-bristle skin brush, which you can buy at a beauty supply, bath shop, or natural-food store.

Once you've disrobed, prop one foot on a stool or tub rim and start by brushing, with circular strokes, up the inside of your raised leg, going from the bottom of the foot to the groin. Then brush up the inside again, using short upward sweeping strokes, two times. Next, do the same (one time circular strokes and twice with sweeping strokes) starting at the top of the foot and going up the outside of the leg to the top of the hip; and finally, the same pattern up the back of the leg and over the buttocks. Now do the same for the other leg (sing a song and think happy thoughts as you go!). Then raise an arm and begin with circular strokes going down the arm from the palm of the hand to the lymph glands at the armpit. Do this once and end with sweeping strokes. Repeat for the outside of the arm, going from the back of the hand to the top of the shoulder. End by bending the elbow and sweeping the outer portion of the upper arm to the armpit. Then repeat for the other arm.

Next, starting at the neck, make sweeping strokes down the outside of the neck, upper chest, around the breasts, and over the sternum toward the bellybutton on both sides. Then sweep across the ribs, going from the edge of the back toward your belly. Finally, end with circular strokes going clockwise around the belly. You may also wish to brush your back (using a long-handled brush, of course) or brush your face, for which you can buy a soft-bristle brush. Note that you're always brushing inward toward the center of the body, to the thoracic duct.

Skin brushing is fun and invigorating, and you essentially give yourself a lymphatic massage.

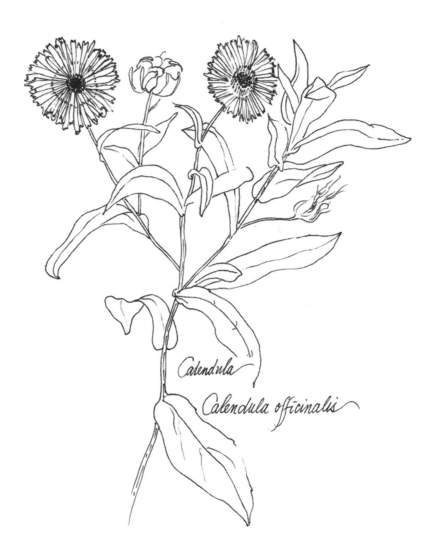

Calendula

Calendula officinalis

Chapter Ten

The Immune System:

Thymus Gland, Spleen, and Community Immunity

Sickness is felt, but health not at all.

Thomas Fuller, M.D.

Nature reveals an immeasurable diversity of individual beings. When you look at a lakeside scene, you see that it's made up of individual trees, grasses, birds, insects, water creatures, and algae. Together all these elements form an ecosystem of individuals concerned with their own survival, yet interacting with each other as a group. If disease sweeps across this scene, it infects not only a few individual plants or animals, but affects a natural community whose overall immunity has been weakened. Our own bodies are the micro-world we each live in, and our immune system is an expression of our relationships within that world and with the world around us — familial, cultural, and global. The alarming increase in cardiovascular, cancer, autoimmune, and environmental illnesses today is an urgent message that we as a species are not managing our relationships with all life in a balanced way.

Thyme
Thymus vulgaris

At its core, the concept of immunity is simple: every second of every day, your body discriminates between what is "you" and "not you." The immune system includes white blood cells (leukocytes) and the lymphoid organs such as the thymus and spleen. It responds to infectious attack or internal mutation in two ways: via nonspecific or innate immunity, and specific or adaptive immunity.

Innate or Nonspecific Immunity

A newborn begins with some innate protection against infection by antibodies introduced through mother's milk, plus the child's own skin, and white blood cells (macrophages and neutrophils, as well as many types of immunoglobulins — primarily IgA) in the mouth, urinary tract, and eye surface.

As a child grows, he or she encounters organisms that overcome the innate system, resulting in sickness. The adaptive or specific immune system is what develops as a result of sickness. Specific antibodies are produced to overcome the invading organism, and the immune system retains the memory of these antibodies so it can rally defenses instantly in future. Most infectious organisms enter the body through the mucosal surfaces in the respiratory, intestinal, and reproductive tracts; therefore, maintaining healthy digestive flora, a slightly alkaline blood pH, and general cleanliness are all key defense strategies.

When innate immunity is triggered, messages are sent to cells throughout the body, usually resulting in inflammation. Swelling traps the healing macrophages and phagocytes, whose job is to engulf intruders and call for help from the adaptive immune system. Phagocytes also release pyrogens, which increase body temperature by producing a fever that speeds up metabolism and the healing process in general. This heat can even directly deactivate some foreign microbes!

Specific or Adaptive Immunity

Cells of the innate immune system influence the adaptive immune system's antibody and T-cell responses. Two types of lymphocytes — B cells (our defense against bacteria) and T cells (defense against viruses, some parasites, and cancer cells) — are at the core of specific immunity. B cells are lymphoid stem cells produced in bone marrow that travel to the spleen and lymph nodes where they mature. B cells produce antibodies called immunoglobulins, each designed to destroy a specific foreign substance known as an antigen. There are five classes of immunoglobulins thus far (there is much still to be understood about our immune system), which include IgA (found mostly in the gut), IgE (linked to hyper allergenic response), and IgG (the most abundant and active type).

T cells are lymphoid cells that travel to the thymus gland, where they develop into mature lymphocytes that circulate between blood and lymph. T cells are covered by surface protein markers, which help identify them to other cells. Each T cell will respond to the body's own cells that have changed in response to invasion or mutation as a result of fighting against fungi, viruses, and cancer cells. There are several types of T cells; first, helper T cells secrete types of interleukin to stimulate the activity of the cytotoxic T cells; second, cytotoxic T cells recognize specific antigens and then inject cytotoxic granules into the targeted cell to destroy it; and third, suppressor T cells shut down the activity of the immune system after infection is cleared. Cytotoxic T cells also attract macrophages to clean up cellular debris, and the resultant waste or mucus is carried away via the lymph system.

The helper T cells have two subclasses — Th1 and Th2, each releasing particular types of interleukins, triggering particular immune functions. One type turns on the inflammatory response; while the other turns it off. Inflammation and autoimmune responses (hypersensitive immune response) are thought to be an imbalance between Th1 and Th2 production.

There's also a fourth type of T cell, the lymphocyte NK or Natural Killer. This T cell destroys cells invaded by viruses or other parasites that have left recognizable antigens on the cell surface. NK cells also destroy cells of tumors or those from transplanted tissues. Finally, interferon is a group of proteins produced naturally by body cells in response to viral infection. It inhibits viral multiplication and increase the activity of NK cells. Listed below are other important members of our immune system.

The Thymus Gland

Our thymus gland is located in the upper chest just behind the sternum and consists of two lobes joining in front of the trachea (see diagram 6, page 194). Both lobes are made up of lymphoid tissue containing tightly packed lymphocytes, epithelium (skin cells), and fat. The thymus gland, which enlarges from about the twelfth week of gestation until puberty, is essential for the maturation of T cells and is a major player in immune response. Forerunner defense cells from the thymus are also sent to the tonsils and the appendix, followed by a hormone that helps the cells to further mature. After puberty and the development of specific immunity, the thymus gland begins to shrink. Lymphoid and epithelial tissues are gradually replaced by fat, though some glandular tissue remains.

In adults, the thymus gland may enlarge if thyroid deficiency, adrenal insufficiency, or spleen deficiency conditions are present, since our thymus has the ability to take over some of the glandular functions of those organs. While modern medicine does not acknowledge the role of the thymus in adulthood, other healing traditions acknowledge activity in this gland throughout life, and practice stimulating it via energy practices such as chi gong and yoga.

Tonsils

"Tonsils" usually refers to the palatine set, a collection of lymphatic tissue located at the back of the throat. Besides producing lymphocytes and monocytes, tonsils contain macrophages that engulf and destroy pathogens entering through the skin. If you feel your immune system may be handicapped due to the removal of tonsils, don't despair. There remain lingual tonsils that lie at the back of the tongue, plus pharyngeal tonsils and adenoids that lie next to the pharynx.

The Spleen

The spleen is found just under the ribs on the left side of the torso (see diagram 6, page 194). It has two primary functions: to remove and destroy worn-out or defective red blood cells approximately 120 days after they have been produced in the bone marrow; and to help fight infection by producing antibodies (phagocytes and lymphocytes) that destroy invading organisms.

In the fetus, the spleen produces red blood cells, but after birth this work is taken up by the bone marrow. Later in life, if our bone marrow is unable to produce red blood cells adequately, as in certain blood diseases, the spleen can again resume some production. Our spleen will enlarge with diseases such as malaria, infectious mononucleosis, schistosomiasis (blood flukes), tuberculosis, typhoid fever, sickle cell anemia, lymphoma, and leukemia. Pain of the spleen can be caused by anything from a severe allergic reaction, to ruptured tissue resulting from a severe blow. Frequent diarrhea is a sign of spleen deficiency. The spleen transforms and replenishes the energy of our blood when we connect to others and the Earth.

Our spleen, pancreas, and liver work as a team to process and distribute nutrients and blood through our bodies; their location at the solar plexus (third chakra or energy center) is connected to the expression of who we are as unique individuals in the world. Note that this is also in the area of the diaphragm — our breath plays an important role, integrating the function of these three important organs.

Supporting our immune system means moving lymphatic fluids as well, since neither system can function without the other. Sustainable immunity requires whole organic foods and vegetable juices, fresh herbs, rest, clean air, exercise (circulation), periodic cleansing of supportive organ systems and their elimination channels, lots of laughter, and making changes that support and enhance the quality of your life.

Herbs that Stimulate and Support Immune Response

Many herbs and foods fall into this category, whether directly antimicrobial, or adaptogenic tonics that strengthen the body as a whole. Below are a few favorites.

Astragalus Root (*Astragalus membranaceus*) The root is widely used in Asia as an immune stimulant, especially for the respiratory and urinary systems. It functions as more of a tonic herb for the adrenal glands, and can be taken for longer periods of time than echinacea.

Blood Root (*Sanguinaria canadensis*) The root is used both externally and internally. Tonic to the lungs, it removes heavy mucus (for pneumonia, combine with wild cherry and mullein), scrofula (lymph nodules / fatty tissue deposits), eczema, ringworm, warts, tumors, and skin cancers. It stimulates bile flow and is diaphoretic, so it's not to be used in cases of acute inflammation. It has some chronic toxicity if used over long periods, so is best used only as needed in combination with other herbs.

Citrus Family Juice, rind, and seeds — especially lemon, blood-orange rind, grapefruit rind, and grapefruit-seed extract — reduce infection and inflammation, remove toxins, stimulate immunity, repel viruses, and help counteract many poisons. Citrus pectin, especially grapefruit pectin, has been shown to activate immunity as well.

Garlic (*Allium sativum*) The raw bulb of garlic, once dubbed "Russian penicillin," is an age-old medicine that does more than dissuade vampires. Research has demonstrated that even the *vapor* of fresh raw garlic "kills bugs dead," including most bacteria, many fungi, and some viruses. It detoxifies the body and protects it against invading microbes, thus is a powerful preventive for virtually any disease or infection.

Goldenseal (*Hydrastis canadensis*) The root and leaf detoxify blood, stimulate immunity, heal mucus membranes, and are very effective for tumors of the female reproductive tract. Use with caution where there is high blood pressure. This herb should not be used more than two weeks continuously since it can inhibit the uptake of B12 in the small intestine. When using this herb, be sure to take acidophilus and eat cultured foods (miso, sauerkraut, rejuvelac).

Indigo Root (*Baptisia tinctoria*) The root stimulates leukocyte production and increases the effectiveness of other immune herbs, especially echinacea. It removes lymph congestion, clears heat and inflammation, and counteracts poisons. It's good for all septic (blood poisoning) conditions, especially when there are putrid, dark secretions. When taken as a tincture, it is a drop-dose herb: 5 – 15 drops every 2 hours. More often it is taken in combination with other herbs or used homeopathically.

Japanese Honeysuckle (*Lonicera japonica*) This plant is easy to cultivate. Its stems and flower buds are sweet and cooling, so useful for lowering fevers, reducing blood pressure, and addressing acute inflammations such as rheumatoid arthritis, mumps, and hepatitis. Honeysuckle is antibacterial, thus effective in treating upper respiratory tract infections, food poisoning, and childhood illnesses. The berries of this plant are poisonous.

Lomatium (*Lomatium dissectum*) The root, also referred to as biscuit root is antiviral, especially for the respiratory system, strep throat, herpes, staphylococcus, tuberculosis, and whooping cough. It's a white blood-cell stimulant and draws up toxins, which it throws out to the skin for elimination. Therefore, combine this herb with blood cleansers such as burdock, yellow dock, or sarsaparilla to avoid rashes. It inhibits gram-positive bacteria and is excellent for flu.

Neem (*Azadirachta indica*) The leaf, bark, and seed of this tree, dubbed the "village pharmacy" in its native India, is a bold blood tonic and immunomodulator. It increases phagocyte and macrophage activity and the number of white blood cells. Neem is antimicrobial and anti-fungal, thus useful for treating skin and dental conditions. Neem leaf helps stabilize blood sugar and strengthen overall immunity, while a tincture or maceration of the oily seed is effective against food poisoning and hepatitis A.

Oregano (*Origanum vulgare*) The oils in the leaves and stem, particularly those grown in the Mediterranean or very hot and dry climates where oils condense, are extremely antimicrobial and anti-fungal. For preventive care, use often as a culinary herb or add to teas. Take the pure essential oil internally (in capsules or drops added to part of a tincture) between meals for fungal and parasite infestations, persistent viral infections, or food poisoning. Pure oregano oil is too strong for ingestion by small children.

Propolis A sticky substance is made from tree resins gathered by bees from cottonwood, pine, fir, and poplar buds in early spring. Bees use it as a cement at the entrance to their hive for fortification and protection. Propolis can be collected in early spring by gathering the fresh, sticky buds that fall from the trees. It is antiviral, antifungal, antibacterial, and can seal and protect the gums and throat, and minor cuts and abrasions to skin.

Shiitake (*Lentinula edodes*), Reishi (*Ganoderma lucidum*), Maitake (*Grifola frondosa*), Cordyceps (*Cordyceps sinensis*), Turkey Tail (*Trametes versicolor*) These medicinal mushrooms are powerful allies! They inhibit abnormal cell growth associated with tumors and cancers. Since they are fungi, it's especially important to know they were grown in a clean environment. People allergic to common mushrooms, or who have a sensitivity to molds and fungi, may be intolerant of medicinal mushrooms. An immune-stimulating component, beta glucan, is extracted and concentrated from maitake and reishi mushrooms and sold as a supplement. These fungi are complex, however, and have many other positive effects, acting as adaptogens, insulin moderators, and tonics.

Tea Tree (*Melaleuca alternifolia*) The leaves and extracted oils of this plant stimulate immunity, reduce infection, restore nerves, inhibit parasites, and protect cells from radiation. Tea tree is antimicrobial and antifungal, thus useful for colds, flu, fungus, bronchitis, dental infection, and wounds.

Thyme (*Thymus* spp.) The leaf is antiviral and antibacterial, especially as it contains the essential oil thymol. It's especially good for respiratory infections, the onset of colds and flu, oral infections, and fungal over-growth. Use the herb internally as food, tea, or tincture. The essential oil is very volatile and can be misted in a room to prevent the spread of illness. It is best taken in a mouthwash, as steam inhalation for the lungs and sinuses, or applied topically in a carrier oil or bath.

Thuja (*Thuja occidentalis*) The tips of this evergreen shrub contain the volatile oils thymol and thujone, thus are antimicrobial. Thuja helps resolve mucus conditions by removing congestion and discharge of the upper respiratory tract, especially where there is congestive heart failure. It's also helpful for chronic colitis, diarrhea, clearing decay in tissue repair, and reducing inflammation. Thuja lessens cysts, tumors, polyps, warts, fungus, and herpes. Use internally and topically for periods of no more than three weeks at a time, though homeopathic thuja can be used for longer periods.

Yerba Mansa (*Anemopsis californica*) The root also contains thymol, so is antibacterial, antifungal, and anti-inflammatory. It can be used for all slow-healing wounds, bleeding, cystitis, ulcers, dental infections, syphilis, and cancers, especially cancer of the uterus. Whether applied externally or taken internally, it's considered an all-round body remedy.

Primary Protection:
The Evolution of Intestinal Flora

When an infant passes through the birth canal, it picks up a host of beneficial bacterial organisms essential to human function. These get into the mouth and down into the intestines and establish the first flora. Mother's milk contains the right ingredients to nourish first flora. *General health of the mother is primary* — especially throughout nursing.

The next floral boost comes from soil microbes (usually via lactate-fermented vegetables like sauerkraut, umeboshi plum, yogurt, real pickles) that assist our digestion, enzyme production and the production of B vitamins. There are up to one thousand billion beneficial microorganisms (four to five pounds worth!) in our large intestine nourishing and sustaining us! These sensitive organisms are easily killed off by chemicals and radiation. Most important, our intestines provide the perfect environment for the production of immune cells, since *70 to 80 percent of our basic immune cells develop there.*

The immune system is a complex multilayered system. Defense mechanisms exist in every part of the body from sebaceous glands in the skin to the marrow of bone. Our body will resist from the outside layers of skin first, then the internal skin of the intestinal tract second. There are three major mid-level immune system lymph aggregations that halt the penetration of microbes: tonsils (and adenoids), Pyor's patches in the small intestinal wall, and the appendix. By the time we have contracted an acute illness, pathogens have passed through half our outer defense layers to the midway point. In chronic illness, pathogens have finally penetrated the deepest layers of our system. Keeping deep layers strong is vital, but so are preventive practices, such as washing hands to reduce exposure to contaminants, breathing fresh air to clear the lungs and dressing warmly when conditions are cold and damp.

Community Immunity

Evolution of humans and disease has shown that improvements in environmental conditions, proper nutrition, good hygiene and sanitation, and quality food and water supplies, have significantly reduced the number of deaths caused by common diseases. These changes, along with a supportive family or extended family network, an honored spiritual life, connection to nature, and using plants as medicine, support the greatest immunity for any community. We are here because our ancestors long before moved toward these changes.

Unfortunately, much of our innate understanding of plants has been lost in the race to modernize life. While current pharmaceutical drugs work quickly, there is a hidden cost to wellness. The frequent use of vaccinations, antibiotics, and synthetic hormones, by even a few, affects all members of a community. These synthetic substances do not decompose, but are flushed into water systems where they affect other living things; for example, killing some bacteria and leaving others that become resistant.

The residue of all chemicals makes its way to our water systems and our food chain. This chemical residue ends up in our blood, and is highly toxic and weakening to our body's defense system. Not only has the wide use of pharmaceuticals caused a marked increase in viral mutations and resistant bacteria for which we have no antidote, but *their improper use results in an estimated*

200,000 deaths per year in the USA, 155,000 of them in hospitals alone!

The common attitude of a "warfare on germs," and subsequent use of medical artillery, pushes pathogens to evolve quickly and aggressively in order to survive. The indiscriminate administration of antibiotics is killing off our natural allies (beneficial bacteria) and crippling our immune systems, jeopardizing the health of our communities. In an effort to remedy this situation in Iceland, for example, the use of antibiotics was drastically reduced for three years, resulting in a 40 percent drop of drug-resistant strains of pathogens. Nature evolves to match the challenges in its environment and is extremely energy efficient. We must question our own efficiency and whether it's worthy to continue an "arms race" with pathogens when we're destroying the planet and ourselves in the process.

Are we appropriate with the use of *our* energy? The time and place for the use of pharmaceutical drugs is only in true need or emergency — using them discriminatingly will insure their effectiveness for those times.

Ways to Boost Immunity

❋ Vitamins are enzymes of living tissues — *eat live, vibrant foods!*

❋ *Reduce our chemical and electromagnetic load* as much as possible by carefully choosing what tools we use and how often we use them.

❋ Eat organic food, limit our intake of sweets, avoid consuming bleached cane sugar, bleached flour, and processed foods.

❋ *Learn our local herbs and eat medicinal herbs common to where we live.* Eat locally produced foods whenever possible. *Use adaptogenic herbs daily;* these help us adapt to stress and strengthen constitutional weaknesses. They have a wide range of beneficial actions, produce no side effects, and restore and maintain balance of biorhythms and help eliminate wastes. Examples are: eleuthero, burdock root, apple, grapeseed, medicinal mushrooms, schizandra berry, suma, licorice root, ashwaganda root, wild oats, dandelion, nettle, citrus peel, pine needles, rosemary, pau d'arco bark, elderberry, ginger, rosehip, plantain leaf, maca root, and wild berries, to name a few.

❊ *Use essential oils!* Oils come from both the immune system and hormonal system of plants, and we have evolved with them. Quality essential oils are extremely powerful allies. Make a spray bottle of strong essential oils in water and mist away!

❊ *Get plenty of fresh air and exercise* every day. Breathe!

❊ *Keep your bowel happy* by cleansing it twice a year and supporting its flora and fauna with foods, herbs, and fiber.

❊ *Cleanse the lymph, liver and kidneys annually.*

❊ *Don't forget energy medicine!* Flower remedies are effective, particularly for children. We are vibrational beings as well as physical ones. There are many integrative therapies for the energy body that are supportive to the immune system.

❊ *Let go of what's not needed*, including unnecessary stuff, destructive habits, unhealthy relationships or living situations in your life.

❊ *Make a "Wellness Soup"* once a week, especially during the winter (recipe below).

❊ *Drink plenty of fresh clean water daily—at least half a gallon (or two liters) a day.*

❊ *Slow down and relax*—take quiet time for yourself.

❊ *Love yourself, love others, love the earth, and keep a peaceful heart.* Love and gratitude enrich and strengthen us.

There are many versions of *Wellness Soup;* here's one:

Wellness Soup

Bring to a boil 2 – 3 quarts of water, turn down to a simmer, and add:

2 large red onions, chopped	2 codonopsis roots, cut
2 large reishi mushrooms, broken	5 jujube dates
1 bulb of garlic, chopped	5 – 10 shiitake mushrooms, sliced
2 tbs. grated ginger	1 large burdock root, sliced
2 tbs. seaweed	leafy greens and root veggies
3 sticks of astragalus root	lotus root when available
2 cups aduki beans	2 – 4 slices of eleuthero root
1 cup of barley	1 – 2 bay leaves

Simmer, covered, for 1½ hours. After removing the soup from heat, add 1 – 2 tablespoons of organic miso and a bit of umeboshi plum if desired. Before serving, remove the reishi mushrooms, eleuthero, astragalus, and codonopsis roots. Add horseradish and / or cayenne pepper to taste. To make this soup as a recuperative broth, omit the aduki beans, simmer more strongly, then strain completely and just drink the broth after adding miso, umeboshi plum, and any hot spices.

Managing Acute Illness

In deciding how to treat an illness, determine whether the symptoms are acute or chronic. "Acute" refers to illnesses of sudden onset and brief duration. They are of high intensity, with severe but short-term symptoms, appearing as colds, flu, and most childhood illnesses. Acute illness needs to be attended to immediately and vigorously. At the first signs, whether swollen glands, sore throat, fever, or fatigue, it's important to quickly assist immune response by reducing the consumption of food — sip on smoothies, vegetable juices, teas, soups and broths, and lots of water. Digestion of heavier foods takes energy away from the immune system. Support fevers instead of derailing them with over-the-counter drugs. Fevers are valuable because they speed up immune response and are safe if carefully monitored, but do not exceed 104°F for more than three days in an adult.

If you feel the need to bring a fever down, wrap your lower legs and feet with ice-cold wet cloths to pull heat away from your head. Use immune-boosting tinctures abundantly (by the teaspoon every two to three hours for adults). Replace water and electrolytes by drinking plenty of water and potassium broth with sea vegetables, nibbling on seaweeds, misting the skin with kelp tea and lavender, or drinking *electro-lemonade* (water with lemon juice, sea salt, and raw honey). Eat plenty of raw garlic, ginger, and cayenne. Sweat and rest! Try the following teas; choose one and drink six cups a day while ill, and up to two cups a day for a week afterward.

 # Immuni-Tea

2 parts each: echinacea leaf / flower, and boneset

1 part each: elderberry, elder flower, chrysanthemum flower, calendula, hibiscus, peppermint, and red raspberry leaf

½ part each: thyme, oregano, and anise seed

¼ part licorice root

Steep longer (2 – 4 hours) for a strong infusion.

Body-boost Decoction

2 parts reishi mushroom

1 part each: pau d'arco, astragalus, cinnamon, cascara sagrada*, licorice, eleuthero, juniper berry, lomatium, and yerba mansa

½ part each: ginger, clove, and allspice

* *Omit cascara sagrada if you have loose stools.*

Simmer, covered, for 30 minutes.

Managing Chronic Illness

Chronic illness is a state of prolonged or recurring disease symptoms. Chronic conditions are harder to treat because they often derive from acute illness, trauma, or toxic exposure that has penetrated deeply into the body over time, resulting in a general systems imbalance. Untreated chronic conditions lead to serious imbalances: degeneration of connective tissues, degeneration of the nervous system, or cancer due to years of cumulative effects from exposure to carcinogens. Treatment for chronic illness requires carefully peeling away symptoms through systematic and thorough cleansing of the body, while building and strengthening organs and nerves and balancing glandular function. Imbalances of the hormonal system or nervous system due to prolonged stress can also lead to chronic illness.

Herring's Law of Cure states, "All cure starts from within and goes out, and from the head down, in reverse order as symptoms have appeared." This implies that when cleansing takes place, symptoms of earlier illnesses or imbalances that contributed to the current state can be briefly relived, from most recent symptoms to the earliest childhood symptoms. "Symptoms" may be both physical (sudden rashes or miniature versions of acute illness) and psychological (suppressed emotions, flashbacks, dreams, and visions).

Due to the possible intensity of this peeling process, it's important to be under the guidance of a professional and to have some kind of social support nearby. In this regard, herbal treatments must always include other healing modalities such as bodywork, acupuncture emotional / movement therapies, and energy medicine (flower remedies, reiki, or other energy work). While the task may seem arduous, healing can be much quicker than the time it took to reach the chronic state. With courage and perseverance, the rewards are the beauty of increased wellness and reconnection of body and spirit — even if the illness is not completely eliminated.

A word about cancer

Cancer is defined as abnormal (damaged DNA) tissue that grows more rapidly than normal tissue and continues growing even after cessation of the stimuli that initiated the growth. Lacking in structural organization and coordination with surrounding tissue, these abnormal cells are considered cancerous if they are malignant. Cancer has been around to some degree for a long time — evidence of bone cancer has been found in million-year-old dinosaur fossils. Today, cancer is a common cause of death worldwide, afflicting all age groups and many other species of animals. Never before has the planet held so many carcinogenic substances — most of them produced by humans. Stopping or reducing the use of and exposure to known carcinogens, along with making economic choices that end their production, is an important part of preventing the risk of cancer now and in the future. Regular cleansing of bowel, liver, and lymph, is imperative for preventing the accumulation of carcinogenic substances in our body.

Herbal treatments for cancer and other serious illnesses have always existed and still remain relevant and important, even in light of modern medicine's progress in bringing about cancer survival in a meaningful way. Herbs, foods, and natural healing methods can be used along with conventional medical treatments to reduce toxification of tissues and strengthen and support all organs. As mentioned previously, some herbs have good reputations for treating cancers, but must be used responsibly, preferably with professional assistance. Famous formulas that have been used successfully in cancer treatment and support include Essiac Formula, Black Salve, Hoxsey Formula, and Scudder's Compound. There are excellent books on herbal approaches to cancer treatment (see references).

Cancer takes years to manifest as obvious symptoms in the body. Many people have an intuitive sense that something is out of balance in their lives and their health — as if something is lurking in the shadows — well before diagnosis. It's important to listen to and explore early warning signs whenever possible. Above all, cancer demands that we face our fear of death and gather our personal power in order to participate immediately in our own well-being on all levels — body, mind and spirit. This takes courage, plus support from family, friends, and one's community. Such connections with self and others are some of the healing gifts of this challenging journey.

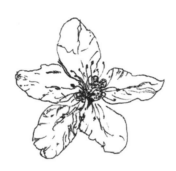

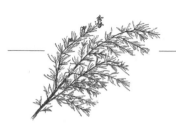

Ten Basic Herbal Actions

1. Alterative – Herbs used to alter the existing nutritive and excretory processes and gradually restore normal body functions (i.e., burdock, chickweed, red raspberry, yellow dock).

2. Astringent – Herbs that pull tissues together, and thus have a toning effect and arrest discharges (i.e., Oregon grape root, oak bark, sage, lemon, and herbs high in tannins).

3. Bitters – Herbs that have a bitter taste and are stimulating tonics to the gastrointestinal mucous membranes (i.e., artichoke, gentian, dandelion, chicory root, mugwort, wormwood).

4. Demulcents – Herbs having mucilaginous properties, which are soothing and protective internally to irritated and inflamed tissues (i.e., licorice, marshmallow, flaxseed, corn silk, slippery elm).

5. Diaphoretic – Herbs that produce perspiration and increased elimination through the skin (i.e., ginger, cayenne, boneset, mint, yarrow).

6. Hepatics – Herbs used to strengthen, tone, and stimulate the secretive functions of the liver, causing an increased flow of bile (i.e., olive, sorrel, wild yam, sarsaparilla, milk thistle, red clover).

7. Nervines – Herbs that are used to balance, restore, and heal the nervous system (i.e., chamomile, lemon balm, lavender, basil, skullcap, oatstraw, passionflower, St. John's wort).

8. Styptics – Herbs that constrict the blood vessels when applied to an external surface or taken internally, and thereby arrest local bleeding or hemorrhaging (i.e., cayenne, plantain, yarrow, shepherd's purse).

9. Tonics – Herbs that stimulate nutrition and permanently increase system tone, energy, and strength (i.e., ginsengs, burdock, nettles, schizandra berry, green grasses).

10. Vermifuges or **anthelminthics** – Herbs used to kill and expel intestinal parasites (i.e., clove, melon seed, wormwood, quassia).

Appendix B

Kitchen Pharmacy Herbs

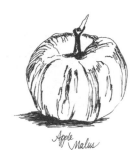

Food is our medicine and kitchen herbs and spices have wonderful healing effects on the body, so use them freely! Here are some of the amazing actions of household herbs:

Aniseed (*Pimpinella anisum*) is excellent for breaking up mucus in the body, relieves cramping in the bowels, and treats colic and flatulence. It is also calming and soothing for the nervous system, so helps in sleeplessness and travel sickness.

Basil (*Ocimum basilicum*) helps balance the nervous system and boosts immunity. It also relaxes the smooth muscles of the digestive system.

Caraway (*Carum carvi*) is an excellent aid to digestion, especially fats, thus it relieves indigestion. Also, it helps ease uterine cramps and stimulates the flow of breast milk.

Cardamom (*Elettaria cardamomum*) warms the body and is useful for indigestion and flatulence. It also resolves excess mucus in the lungs and restores nerves.

Cayenne (*Capsicum* sp.) is the best food for the circulatory system. It raises or lowers blood pressure as needed by helping the vessels gain elasticity. Used raw, it rebuilds tissue in the stomach and heals ulcers (the opposite is true of cooked chilies). It aids elimination and perspiration and can be used to stop wounds from bleeding.

Celery Seed (*Apium graveolens*) is a sedative for the nerves, but also helps heal bronchitis, gout and rheumatic conditions.

Chervil (*Anthriscus cerefolium*) can be used to lower blood pressure. The fresh-pressed flowering herb is used for eczema, abscesses, and general blood cleansing.

Chive (*Allium schoenoprasum*) is stimulating to the appetite and promotes digestion. The onion family generally supports the immune system, but chive is highest in iron.

Cinnamon (*Cinnamomum zeylanicum*) is warming and a good tonic for stomachaches, sugar metabolism, and lung congestion. It also eases nausea, flatulence, and diarrhea.

Clove (*Eugenia caryophyllata*) increases circulation, promotes digestion, decreases nausea and vomiting, and clears mucus (allspice acts similarly). Clove is capable of inhibiting fungi and viruses, thus is used to treat parasites and tooth decay.

Coriander (*Coriandrum sativum*) has a cooling effect on the body. It is antispasmodic, and the essential oil can be applied externally to painful joints.

Cumin (*Cuminum cyminum*) is cooling to the digestive tract and calms flatulence. It is also a tonic herb for the heart and uterus.

Fennel (*Foeniculum vulgare*) has a warming effect and aids digestion by increasing the metabolic processes in general. It helps dissolve and disperse mucus and fats, and has estrogenic-like properties that promote the flow of breast milk and menses.

Fenugreek (*Trigonella foenum-graecum*) contains plant steroids that help balance the pancreas (blood sugar), soothe ulcerated stomachs, increase breast milk, and build the body (helps in weight / mass gain).

Garlic (*Allium sativum*) is the ultimate blood cleanser (cooked or raw) and natural antibiotic (raw only). The fresh juice is also effective for cramps, spasms, and seizures. It lowers blood pressure and reduces clot / platelet aggregation within blood vessels. It is an antioxidant and stimulant to the immune system.

Ginger (*Zingiber officinale*) is a versatile stimulant and diaphoretic. Its dispersing effect enhances the use of other herbs. Not to be taken with high blood pressure or in cases of extreme inflammation of the liver or overly dry skin.

Marjoram (*Origanum majorana*) is both a stimulant and relaxant. It is antiseptic and promotes digestion. Both marjoram and its cousin, oregano

(*Origanum vulgare*), expel mucus, ease cramps, and soothe the bowels. Oregano is a powerful antiviral.

Mustard Seed (*Brassica alba, nigra* and other sp.) is a blood cleanser and stimulates the skin. It is warming, opens the solar plexus, and aids in food assimilation.

Nutmeg and Mace (*Myristica fragrans*) — A strong stimulant to the nervous system, nutmeg helps mitigate the chemical effects of coffee and encourages menses. Mace is the outer covering of the nutmeg, and has a more antiseptic action.

Parsley, curly or Italian (*Petroselium* sp.) has a very high vitamin and mineral content and is rich in chlorophyll. Excellent for countering anemia, it is a blood cleanser, promotes menses, and reduces production of large amounts of breast milk.

Pepper (*Piper nigrum*) should always be freshly ground and added *after* cooking. It is a natural preservative, antifungal, antibacterial, expels mucus, and stimulates the colon.

Rosemary (*Rosmarinus officinalis*) is useful for indigestion, colic, nausea, flatulence, and nervousness. It stimulates and nourishes the brain and lungs and is high in calcium and antioxidants.

Sage (*Salvia officinalis*) is a muscle relaxant, antiseptic, and astringent, and helps slow fluid secretions (perspiration, vaginal discharge, and breast milk, etc.). It makes a good gargle.

Thyme (*Thymus vulgare*) is one of the strongest antimicrobial herbs, as it activates and strengthens the immune system. In excessive amounts it can cause depression.

Turmeric (*Curcuma longa*) is a strong blood and liver cleanser, and is an effective antioxidant and strong anti-inflammatory.

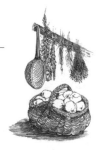

Kitchen Pharmacy Recipes

Barley Water

Barley water is an excellent kidney tonic, especially in cold weather. Simply rinse one-fourth cup whole unpearled barley and put in a saucer with 2 cups of water. Add a little grated ginger and / or lemon peel, cover the pot, and simmer, low, for 20 minutes. Strain off the water and sip as a tea, adding maple syrup or molasses if desired.

Elderberry Blast!

A great way to get a daily dose of this powerful immune-stimulating herb! Fill a jar halfway with dried or fresh elderberries, and pour in raw apple cider vinegar to the top. Cap tightly and store in a dark place for 2 weeks, shaking the jar occasionally. Pour off the berry vinegar and store in another jar. Add more vinegar to make another batch with the same berries — you can repeat this up to 4 times with dried berries or twice with fresh ones. Use in the Good Mornin' Drink below.

Good Mornin' Drink

Using a generous mug, fill to one third with organic apple juice, add 1 to 2 teaspoons of elderberry vinegar, one to two droppers full of super-tonic, and 1 teaspoon of plain apple cider vinegar. Fill the rest of the mug with boiled water and sit down to slowly sip in the dawn of day. The malic acid in this beverage will balance stomach acids and stimulate enzyme activity. It also stimulates immunity and circulation, and gently opens the bowels while flushing the kidneys.

Marinated Garlic

Marinated garlic is much less odorous than its fresh, raw counterpart, but unlike cooked garlic, its antimicrobial action remains intact. There are as many recipes as there are countries, but here's a tasty one from James Green (see references) that will delight even the most staunch "never raw garlic" person! Combine the following in a glass jar and cap tightly: 1 cup fresh, peeled, whole organic garlic cloves, ½ cup Bragg Liquid Aminos or tamari sauce, ½ cup raw honey, ½ cup pure water, plus any other spices or lemon as you wish. Place in the refrigerator and let it age for at least 1 month (the longer, the less of a sting). Eat 2 or 3 cloves per day. Another tasty version is to fill a jar with peeled garlic cloves, whole or sliced. Pour honey into the jar to halfway, then fill to the top with fresh-squeezed lemon juice. Mix well. Place a thick slice of lemon on top to keep the garlic down, and refrigerate to marinate at least one month.

Potassium Broth

For fevers, flu, colds, and recovery from general depletion, nothing picks up tissues like a good potassium broth. Take out your biggest pot (a pasta pot with removable strainer works best, since you can just lift out the vegetables after cooking). Clean and coarsely cut up these potassium / electrolyte-rich vegetables: ¼ part onions and garlic, ¼ part potato peelings, ¼ part carrots and beets, and ¼ part greens (kale, collards, nettle, chard, celery.), plus any herbs or spices (seaweed, thyme, oregano, basil, cilantro, rosemary, ginger, cumin, fennel, marjoram, celery seed), or medicinal mushrooms. Bring to a boil and cover. Simmer, very low, for 2 hours, then strain off the broth, which can be stored for up to three days in the refrigerator, or for months in the freezer.

Rejuvelac (homemade intestinal flora)

Rejuvelac contains B-complex vitamins including B12, plus vitamins K and E, in addition to lactic acid and water-soluble minerals. Good rejuvelac has a somewhat lemony and sour flavor. Use organic whole wheat, millet, rye, oats, brown rice, and barley, and season with herbs if you desire. Always rinse the grains first, before soaking them. In a sterilized jar, cover 1 cup of grain with 2 – 4 cups purified water. Allow to soak for 24 hours, covered, in a warm place (60 – 80°F / 30°C) to ferment.

The rejuvelac is the water left after this process. Strain off the water and refrigerate. Drink up to 2 cups daily, adding lemon for flavor. It can also be added to recipes. Rinse grains and then add the same amount of water to repeat the process with the same grains — they can be reused 3 to 5 times.

Sauerkraut

Some very good, organic, live-cultured brands of sauerkraut are on the market, but making your own is easy and fun! There are various recipes and it can take a few batches to perfect, but the basic ingredients are organic raw shredded cabbage, herbs and spices, salt and / or tamari, and whey if desired. Use a stone crock jar with fitted lid, or glass jar with fitted lid (you can also use a plate and weight to hold it down firmly on the cabbage). Sterilize the jar with boiling water and dry thoroughly. Knead salt (1 to 2 teaspoons for every 4 cups of cabbage) into cabbage until it starts releasing its juices — about 10 to 15 minutes.

Then mix in additions as desired: seaweeds, seeds (cumin, caraway, coriander, or celery), and herbs (thyme, marjoram, turmeric, ginger, or juniper), and even other vegetables such as shredded carrot. Some people like to add 1 tsp. powdered goat whey or liquid whey from yogurt to speed up the souring process.

Toss well, pack down in jar, and cover the top with outer cabbage leaves. Weigh lid down with a stone and let sit at room temperature (70 – 80°F / 35°C) for 3 to 4 days, then place jar in the refrigerator to sour for up to another month before eating (you can also let it ferment for 1 month at a cool room temperature).

Sauerkraut will keep in the fridge for a very long time and will continue to slowly ripen. Take 1 heaping tablespoon per day before a meal.

Sunflower Sauce

Simply puree any amount of organic sunflower seed kernels (just the meats) in twice the amount of spring or distilled water. Pour into a glass jar or ceramic container with glass lid and place on a warm, sunny windowsill for about 6 hours. When you see bubbling, it means the organisms are happily dancing, so slow down the party by putting the container in the refrigerator. Use the sauce for making salad dressings, veggie sauces, or smoothies for up to 3 days, then start a new batch!

Super-tonic

Make a quart of this in autumn and use it through the winter to keep your immune system boosted. In a good blender, combine ¼ part peeled and chopped fresh horseradish root, ¼ part red onion, ¼ part peeled garlic, and ¼ part ginger and fresh hot chilies (jalapeño, serrano, or habañero, depending on how hot you can handle it). Additionally, any strong immune herbs such as oregano, thyme, or rosemary can be added. Fill to the top (cover) with organic, raw apple cider vinegar and blend it just enough so it pours easily into a glass jar.

Seal in a glass jar and keep in the dark for 2 to 4 weeks (the longer the better), then strain mixture through a colander lined with cheesecloth. Take up the ends of the cloth and squeeze out excess liquid (*use gloves* if your mixture contains very hot chilies!).

Keep some out in the kitchen in a dropper container or vinegar dispenser; store the remainder in a cool, dark place (a brown glass bottle works best). Use as a condiment on salads and stir-fry, or drink in warm water. Take it along when you travel, and add it to apple juice.

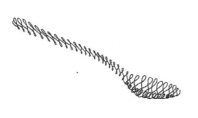

Determining Dosage

Dosage of herbs is variable, since it is influenced by a person's age, body weight, and individual sensitivity to the plants, plus the quality and strength of the herbal preparation used. It's important to follow body wisdom by starting with lower dosages and then increasing them to the standard dose, assuming no symptoms of sensitivity (rash, hives, abdominal, liver, or kidney pain, or insomnia, etc.) develop.

The adult standard dose for *most* (but not all) herbs is 3 cups of infusion or decoction a day, which is equivalent to 6 "00" capsules per day, or 3 teaspoons (40+ drops per teaspoon, depending on dropper size) of tincture each day. In general, very acrid, bitter, or pungent herbs have stronger essential oils and can be taken in smaller amounts. Six to eight cups a day can be consumed of *tonic* infusions and decoctions. If one is very ill, all dosages can be increased, depending on the individual.

Dosages recommended for children

Infants under one year can use normal infusion strength, introduce ½ teaspoon (this can be further diluted in water or milk). Wait 30 minutes and monitor for any adverse reactions. Then, give one teaspoon of infusion 3 to 6 times per day, not exceeding half a cup of infusion.

Children 1 – 3 years old can have 2 tablespoons of infusion or decoction up to 6 times per day. They can also have herbal glycerate tinctures based on body weight (see Clark's rule below). Introducing herbs into the bath is excellent for infants and children.

Children 3 – 12 years can have up to ½ cup of tea 3 to 4 times per day (maximum 2 cups) and can take up to 2 teaspoons tincture per day in ½-teaspoon increments. If the herbs are tinctured in alcohol, mix dosage with a small amount of just-boiled water and allow to cool so alcohol dissipates. Again, it's best to start with low dosages, since this depends on general health, the child's body weight, and the type of herb taken.

Clark's Rule for determining dosage is to divide body weight in pounds by 150. The resultant fraction or percentage will indicate the correct dose. So while for a child of 75 lb. would require 50 percent of a standard dose, an adult of 120 lb. would need 80 percent. Usually, an adult under 100 lb. in weight would find two teaspoons of tincture a day enough, yet could consume three to four cups tea. From 100 – 130 lb., take two teaspoons. a day to start, then increase to three teaspoons. Someone over 130 lb. can normally take up to 4 to 6 teaspoons of tincture per day and up to 6 cups of tea. Some commercial preparations are quite weak and dosage may be practically doubled, while some homemade preparations are strong and can be reduced.

There are times when the synergistic energy of the herb is all that's needed, in which case, *less is more.* If you feel intuitively aligned with a particular herb, you may choose to simply take 10 drops or less at a time to affect the subtle body in a way similar to flower remedies and homeopathy.

Drop-dose Herbs are potentially toxic when taken internally; they have very strong alkaloids and strong medicinal action, so are taken by the drop in doses that usually do not exceed 15 drops 2 to 6 times a day. Examples: arnica, wild indigo, lobelia, chaparral, pokeroot, and ipecacuanha.

In all cases, when taking herbs (or anything for that matter) *listen to your intuition and your body!* Every-body is unique, and, ultimately, the natural intelligence of your body (body wisdom) knows exactly what's needed to assist the healing process. The more you open to dialogue with your body, the more appropriately and efficiently you can take of yourself. Even the most competent practitioner can't fully know what *you* need.

About Echinacea (Cone flower)

All nine species of echinacea are detoxifying and immune stimulating, though *E. angustifolia*, *E. purpurea*, and *E. pallida* are most commonly used. The key constituents that are antibacterial and antiviral cause a tingling sensation on the tongue. It also has polysaccharides, which are anti-inflammatory and stimulate production of interferon (a protein that inhibits virus replication). Echinacea strengthens blood vessels and is strongly antioxidant. It was traditionally used for snakebite and other wounds because it effectively reduces poisons in the system.

Echinacea boosts the immune system by increasing the number and activity of white blood cells and hastening their ability to recognize pathogens. It does this by stimulating the production of alpha 1 and alpha 2 gammaglobulin cells (found primarily in the liver) and increasing the body's production of killer T cells. It also protects healthy cells during an infection. It normally takes four to five days for the body to recognize and produce antibodies for a newly introduced pathogen, but using echinacea will speed that process considerably. Timely and frequent administration of a high-quality echinacea preparation can boost the immune system to prevent the onset of symptoms, reduce their intensity, and reduce infection.

Suggested Adult Dosages of High-quality Echinacea Tincture

Tonic dose: 10 drops a day of tincture for up to 9 months.

Maintenance dose: 20 drops of tincture, twice a day for up to 2 months.

Protective dose: 40 – 60 drops 3 times a day for 10 days; rest 4 days, repeat if needed.

Full course: For countering acute conditions such as viral infection that can lead to chronic illness, use 40 drops every 2 waking hours for 5 to 10 days, then go to protective dose. Combine with other antiviral herbs / oils.

Echinacea is contraindicated for those with very high white blood-cell counts, for example, with leukemia. A maintenance dose should be taken if you're on a cleanse. If you feel the first signs of cold / flu, then it's most effective to take 20 drops every hour for the first 12 hours before using the protective dose.

Suggested doses for children

Children under 6 years can be given 10 drops a day a little at a time.

Children 7 – 10 years can take 20 drops a day.

Children 11 – 13 years can take 30 – 50 drops a day.

These recommendations are for strong, high-quality organic tinctures and should always be accompanied by a wholesome (no sugar, no caffeine, no junk-food) diet and plenty of fresh water.

Herbal First-aid Kit

In addition to a good conventional first-aid kit (bandages, scissors, tweezers, and tape, etc.), there are various herbal formulas that are easy to apply and effective in emergency situations. Below is a list of those to include in your home, travel, and car kits.

Rescue Remedy or other Flower Remedy drops – Use for shock, trauma, or headache, can be applied internally or externally to injured area. A Rescue Remedy cream is also available.

Lobelia Tincture – Take 5 – 30 drops on tongue or lips for shock, unconsciousness, coma, hysteria, severe cramping, muscle spasm, asthma or anaphylactic shock.

Cayenne Tincture – Take 5 – 40 drops in mouth or on lips for shock, heart attack, stroke, hypothermia, internal bleeding, sleepiness, severe nasal congestion, wound antiseptic.

Emergency Tincture – Combine half cayenne, half lobelia, plus rescue remedy, use this combination for shock, unconsciousness, disorientation, severe bleeding, heart attack, faintness, and stroke.

Echinacea Tincture – Use as needed for onset of illness, snake or spider bite (use both internally and on bite), wound wash, and blood or food poisoning. Use plenty as needed.

Arnica montana – Use as a salve, gel, flower oil, tincture, or the dried herb to make a poultice and apply externally. Used for bruising and jarring of any kind; *not* to be used on open wounds. Homeopathic arnica tablets are taken internally and are very effective.

Lavender Oil – Take for burns, wounds, insect bites, insomnia, and nervousness. Lavender oil can be applied directly on the skin, mixed with carrier oils, or used in poultices. A good burn poultice is made from lavender oil mixed in wheat germ, raw honey, and vitamin E. Just add lavender to wet bentonite clay for insect bites.

Tea Tree Oil – Use for wounds, fungus, mouth infection (mouthwash), and fleas. A nice bug repellent includes lavender, tea tree, rosemary, citronella or lemon grass, peppermint, and thyme essential oils in a carrier oil (jojoba, almond, grape seed) or spray.

Whole Cloves or Tincture of Clove – Use for toothache, gargle, wounds, and intestinal parasites.

Whole Juniper Berries – Make a tea for severe edema, kidney / bladder infection, and digestive upset.

Slippery Elm Bark Powder – Use for making poultices, good for ulcers or irritated stomach, coughing, sore throat, bronchitis, and promoting nourishment. Also for making herbal casts.

Fresh bulb of Garlic – Use for poultices, intestinal parasites, and all bacterial and viral infections.

Wheat Germ Oil or Vitamin E Capsules – Use for burns and poultice making for anti-scarring.

St. John's Wort Oil – Use for trauma and infections (internal or external), burns, and muscle cramps.

Yarrow Leaf and Flower – Use for wounds; especially drawing poisons and pus out of the area. It also slows bleeding and can be used for internal hemorrhaging and heavy menstrual bleeding.

Ginger Powder or Pieces – Take for motion sickness, nausea, cold limbs, and indigestion.

Plantain Leaf. Have dried leaf or tincture handy in case fresh is not available. Use for making poultices (bites, stings, cuts, itching) to prevent blood poisoning.

Small Jar of Raw Honey – Use for poultice making, scratchy throat, blood-sugar drop, burn paste.

Aloe Vera – Use for burns and wounds. The fresh leaf is very best, but keep gel on hand.

Bentonite (or green) Clay. Use to draw out poison, tick heads, for poison oak, and for poultice making.

Wound Powder – Combine equal parts of comfrey root powder, goldenseal / barberry or Oregon grape root powder, and marshmallow root powder, plus one part of myrrh, cayenne, and garlic powder combination. This powder can be dusted on wounds or used as an herbal cast with slippery elm. Moisten into a workable paste with purified water, olive oil, and lavender oil and pack into *clean* wound. Alternatively, this combination works well as a thin paste (with water) taken internally for bleeding ulcers and irritable bowel. **Do not** use it for deep puncture wounds.

Cayenne Pepper Powder – The *first* thing to dust on cuts, scrapes, and lacerations to prevent excessive blood loss and infection. Drink up to 1 tsp. cayenne in warm water for bleeding ulcers.

Herbal Wound Salve – Apply for wound healing, diaper rash, hemorrhoids, bites, cuts, and split lips, etc.

Bitter Tonic / Digestive Tincture – All-purpose aid for stomach upset and wound washing.

Grapefruit Seed Extract – Use 5-15 drops in water or juice for intestinal parasites and infections.

Ear Oil – Usually with mullein, St. John's Wort, and garlic in olive oil, ear oil is excellent for ear infection and earache. Be sure to warm it to body temperature and shake well before using.

Herbal Snuff – Combine equal parts of goldenseal (or Oregon grape-root powder), bayberry powder, garlic and cayenne powders. Put a small amount on the back of your hand, and hold one nostril shut as you inhale or "snort" the powder with the other. It also works on scrapes.

Blister Powder – Mix equal parts of powdered myrrh and goldenseal (or Oregon grape root); dust on blisters, especially weeping ones. Also used to prevent infections in second-degree burns.

Organic Coffee Tincture – Take by the dropper-full to combat the effects of nerve poisons (some poisonous mushrooms such as aconite, ingestion of poisonous plants such as hemlock, and the venom of certain snakes and spiders), which cause sudden drowsiness and nervous-system failure. Also use to reduce sleepiness while driving.

References and Suggested Reading

Arvigo, Rosita. *Sastun.* New York, NY: HarperCollins Publishing, 1994.

Barnard, Julian and Martine. *The Healing Herbs of Edward Bach.* Bath, England: Ashgrove Press Ltd., 1988.

Beinfield, Harriet and Efrem Korngold. *Between Heaven and Earth.* New York, NY: Ballantine Books, 1991.

Bown, Deni, ed. *The New Encyclopedia of Herbs and Their Uses* (The Herb Society of America). New York, NY: DK Publishing, 1995, 2001.

Buhner, Stephen Harrod. *Herbal Antibiotics.* North Adams, MA: Storey Publishing, 1999.

Buhner, Stephen Harrod. *Herbs for Hepatitis C.* North Adams, MA: Storey Publishing, 2000.

Chopra, Deepak. *Quantum Healing.* New York, NY: Bantam Books, 1989.

Christopher, David. *Dr. John Raymond Christopher: An Herbal Legacy of Courage.* Springville, UT: Christopher Publications, 1993.

Christopher, John Raymond. *The School of Natural Healing,* 20th Anniversary ed., Springville, UT: Christopher Publications, 1996.

Cowan, Eliot. *Plant Spirit Medicine.* Newberg, OR: Swan Raven & Co., 1995.

Crawford, Amanda McQuade. *The Herbal Menopause Book.* Freedom, CA: Crossing Press, 1996.

Davis, Jill Rosemary. *Self Heal: The Complete Home Guide to Natural Healing, Herbs Nutrition.* Dublin, Ireland / UK: Newleaf; Gill & Macmillan, 2000.

Eliot, Rose and de Paoli, Carlo. *Kitchen Pharmacy: How to Make Your Own Remedies.* London: Tiger Books International, 1991.

Foster, Steven and Chongxi, Yue. *Herbal Emissaries: Bringing Chinese Herbs to the West.* Rochester, VT: Healing Arts Press, 1992.

Gascoigne, Stephen. *The Manual of Conventional Medicine for Alternative Practitioners.* Surrey, UK: Jigme Press, 1994.

Gershon, M.D., Michael. *The Second Brain.* New York, NY: HarperCollins Publishers, 1998.

Gladstar, Rosemary. *Herbal Healing for Women.* New York, NY: Simon and Schuster, 1993.

Green, James. *The Male Herbal.* Freedom, CA: Crossing Press, 1991.

Green, James. *The Herbal Medicine Maker's Handbook.* Berkeley, CA: Ten Speed Press, 2000.

Grieve, Mrs. M. *A Modern Herbal.* London, England: Penguin Books, Ltd., 1980.

Hobbs, Christopher. *Foundations of Health.* Capitola, CA: Botanica Press, 1992.

Hobbs, Christopher. *Medicinal Mushrooms; An Exploration of Tradition, Healing and Culture.* Summertown, TN: Botanica Press, 1995.

Hobbs, Christopher. *Natural Therapy for Your Liver.* New York, NY: Penguin Putnam, Inc., 1986.

Hoffman, David. *An Elders' Herbal.* Rochester, NY: Healing Arts Press, 1993.

Hoffman, David. *The Complete Illustrated Holistic Herbal.* Element Books Ltd. UK, 1996.

Holmes, Peter. *The Energetics of Western Herbs Volumes I and II.* Berkeley, CA: NatTrop Publishing, 1993.

Jensen, Bernard. *Tissue Cleansing Through Bowel Management.* Escondido, CA: Bernard Jensen Enterprises, 1981.

Kapit, Wynn and Lawrence M. Elson. *The Anatomy Coloring Book.* New York, NY: Harper & Row Publishers, 1977.

Kay, Margarita Artschwager. *Healing with Plants in the American and Mexican West.* Tucson, AZ: The University of Arizona Press, 1996.

Kloss, Jethro. *Back to Eden.* Loma Linda, CA: Back to Eden Books Publishing Co., 1997.

Lad, M.D., Vasant. *Ayurveda; The Science of Self-Healing.* Wilmot, WI: Lotus Press, 1990.

Lappé, Marc and Bailey, Britt. *Against the Grain.* Monroe, ME: Canmar Courage Press, 1998.

Lawless, Julia. *The Encyclopedia of Essential Oils.* Rockport, MA: Element Books, 1992.

Lockie, Dr. Andrew. *The Family Guide to Homeopathy.* New York, NY: Simon and Schuster, 1989.

Lust, John. *The Herb Book.* New York, NY: Benedict Lust Publications/Bantam Books, 1974.

Mabey, Richard, ed. *The New Age Herbalist.* New York, NY: Macmillan Publishing Company, 1988.

Moore, Michael. *Medicinal Plants of the Mountain West.* Santa Fe, NM: The Museum of New Mexico Press, 1979.

Moore, Michael. *Medicinal Plants of the Pacific West.* Santa Fe, NM: Red Crane Press, 1993.

Myss, Caroline, Ph.D. *Anatomy of the Spirit.* New York, NY: Harmony Books, 1996.

Naiman, Ingrid. *Cancer Salves: A Botanical Approach to Treatment.* Santa Fe, NM: Seventh Ray Press, 1999.

Parker, Janet, ed. *Anatomica's Body Atlas.* San Diego, CA: Laurel Glen Publishing, 2002.

Rector-Page, Linda G. *Healthy Healing: An Alternative Healing Reference.* Healthy Healing Publications, 1992.

Schulze, Richard. *Common Sense Health and Healing.* Santa Monica, CA: Natural Healing Publications, 2002.

Smith, Ed. *Therapeutic Herb Manual.* Williams, OR: Ed Smith, 1999.

Stipanuk, Martha H., ed. *Biochemical and Physiological Aspects of Human Nutrition.* Philadelphia, PA: W. B. Saunders Company, 2000.

Tierra, Michael. *Planetary Herbology.* Twin Lakes, WI: Lotus Press, 1988.

Tierra, Michael and Lesley. *Chinese-Plantetary Herbal Diagnosis.* Santa Cruz, CA: Michael and Lesley Tierra, 1988.

Tilford, Gregory L. *Edible and Medicinal Plants of the West.* Missoula, MT: Mountain Press Publishing Co., 1997.

Venables, Betty. *Electromagnetic Radiation and Your Health.* Glebe, NSW, Australia: Fast Books, 1999.

Watson, Brenda. *Renew Your Life.* Clearwater, FL: Renew Life Press, 2002.

Weed, Susan. *Wild Woman Herbal for the Childbearing Year.* Woodstock, NY: Ashtree Publishing, 1986.

White, M.D., Linda B. and Steven Foster. *The Herbal Drugstore.* Rodale Press, 2000.

Willard, Terry, Ph.D. *Textbook of Modern Herbology.* Calgary, Canada: Progressive Publishing, Inc., 1988.

Wood, Matthew. *The Book of Herbal Wisdom: Using Plants as Medicines.* Berkeley, CA: North Atlantic Books, 1997

Wood, Matthew. *The Practice of Traditional Western Herbalism.* Berkeley, CA: North Atlantic Books, 2004.

Yance, Donald R. *Herbal Medicine Healing & Cancer.* Chicago, IL: Keats Publishing, 1999.

American Botanical Pharmacy
800-437-2362
www.herbdoc.com

Gravity-fed Colonic Cleansing
www.Angelfarms.com

Live Food Products
Bragg Apple Cider Vinegar and Liquid Aminos
Santa Barbara, CA 93102
800-446-1990
www.bragg.com

Organic Castor Oil and Personal Care Products
www.ohohorganic.com

Body Pure by HeelBHI
www.heelusa.com

Dr. Schuessler's Biochemic Cell Salts
Via Hylands Homeopathic: www.HylandsStore.com
Via Boiron Homeopathic: www.affordablehomeopathy.com

Manual Lymphatic Drainage Massage Practitioners
www.massage_classifieds.com / manuallymphaticdrainage.htm

Selected Associations

American Botanical Council
http://www.herbalgram.org/

The Herb Society (UK)
www.herbsociety.co.uk

International Aromatherapy and Herb Association
www.aromaherbshow.com

Index

A

abdominal pain, 29–31, 61
acid imbalance, 41–43
adaptogenic herbs, 182
adrenal glands, 114, 136–141, 145, 180
allergies, 139–141
alternative herbs, 231
Alzheimer's disease, 184–185
American Botanical Pharmacy's Intestinal Formulas, 27–28, 34, 61, 249
anemia, 90–91
ANS (autonomic nervous system), 178
anthelminthics (anti-parasitic herbs), 35, 231
anti-lithic herbs, 128
anti-microbial herbs, 197, 201
antidiuretic hormone, 145
antiseptic herbs, 128
anxiety, 185–186
appendix, 29–31, 222
arteriolosclerosis, 92–93, 98
arthritis, 93–94
asthma, 114–117, 243
astringent herbs, 44, 231
atherosclerosis, 81
autonomic nervous system (ANS), 178
Ayurvedic tradition / medicine, 13, 26, 106

B

B cells, 215
Bach flower remedies, 34, 66, 243
backache, 29
bacteria, 15–17, 87, 222–223, 244
baths / showers. *See* hydrotherapy
benign prostate hypertrophy (BPH), 169–170
bentonite clay, 24, 244
bitter tonics, 58, 59, 70, 71, 231, 242, 245
bladder, 133–136

blister powder, 245
blood: anemia, 90–92; arthritis, 93; benefits of bowel cleansing to the, 16; cartilage and healthy, 85; essential fatty acids and, 82; function of the, 75, 77; good dental hygiene essential to, 86; herbs for the, 244; high blood pressure, 98; low blood pressure, 99; skin and cleansing of the, 89
blood poisoning, 244
boils, 7
bones, 77, 85–86, 94, 99–100
bodywork: benefits of, 88; during cleanse, 25, 65, 68, 73, 89; for lymph stimulation, 88; to support connective tissue, 84, 85
bowel: emotions and the, 27, 29, 32; foods for moistening stools, 27; herbs for the, 24–26; influence on the heart, 78; irritable bowel syndrome, 42, 44–45; as partner to the lungs, 111
bowel cleanse: benefits of, 13–14, 16–17; liver cleanse and the, 59, 61, 67; and lymph health, 201, 208; prior to kidney cleanse, 130; process of, 24–29; skin cleanse and, 89; for treating asthma, 114
brain and spinal cord (central nervous system): care under stress, 182–184; concussion, 186–187; depression, 187–188; diagram of the, 176; essential fatty acids and the, 83; function of the, 177–180; headaches and the, 184, 189–190; imbalance, 191
breast-feeding, 157–158
bronchitis, 111, 115–118, 246
bruising, 245
bug repellent, 244
burns, 243-245

C

cancer, 7, 17, 133, 228–229
candida, 29, 44, 165

cardiovascular disease, 78, 81–82, 86, 100–101
cartilage, 77, 83–85
castor oil pack, 8, 249
cataracts, 120–121
central nervous system. *See* brain and spinal cord
chakras, 13, 206–207
cholesterol, 79, 96–97
circulatory system: anemia, 90–92; arteriolosclerosis, 92–93; arthritis, 93–94; bones, 77, 85–86, 94, 99–100; and the brain, 179; cholesterol, 79, 96–97; diagram of lungs and heart, 76; eczema and rashes, 95; emotions and the, 80, 92, 93; essential fatty acids, 82–83; function of the, 75, 77; gout, 96; herbal remedies for the, 23, 80–82, 84–87, 89; high cholesterol, 96–97; hypertension, 98; ligaments, tendons and cartilage, 83–85; low blood pressure, 99; osteoporosis, 99–100; rheumatism, 101; skin, 49, 60, 77, 82, 87–89, 95-96; strokes, 100–101; teeth, 86–87; varicose veins, 102–103. *See also* heart
Clark's Rule, for determining dosage, 240
cleanses. *See* bowel cleanse; detoxification; liver cleanse
CNS. *See* brain and spinal cord
colitis, 31–32
colonic cleansing, 31, 35, 67, 69, 249
compress, 7
concussion, 186–187
congestion, nasal, 244, 245
congestive heart failure (CVD), 78
constipation, 15, 32, 61, 126
coronary, 78, 81–82, 86, 243
coughs, 109, 110, 244
cramps, 150, 243, 244
cuts / scrapes / lacerations, 245
CVD (congestive heart failure), 78
cystic duct, 57

herbal remedies: adaptogenic herbs, 182; for the adrenal glands, 137–138; for alleviating stress / increasing energy, 137–138; alternative herbs, 231; anti-microbial herbs, 197, 201; astringent herbs, 44, 231; basic herbal actions, 231–232; bitter tonics, 58, 59, 70, 71, 231; for the bowel, 24–26; circulatory system, 23, 80–82, 84–87, 89; decoctions, 7, 239; demulcent herbs, 128, 231; determining dosage, 239–241; diaphoretic herbs, 108, 112–113, 197, 231; for the digestive system, 23–24, 41, 48–49, 58–59, 244, 245; diuretic herbs, 126–127, 197; first-aid kit, 243–245; hepatic herbs, 58, 231; for immune response, 24, 218–221; kidney cleanse, 131–133; kitchen pharmacy herbs, 232–234; liver flush, 59, 63–65; for the lungs, 109–114; for men, 168–169; nervines, 166, 167, 231; nervous system, 180–182, 245, 247; primary lymph herbs, 197–200; relaxants, 181; respiratory system, 23, 106–109, 244; stimulants, 180–181; styptics, 232; tonics, 7, 232, 241; urinary system, 24, 98, 126–130, 133–136, 244; vermifuges, 35, 232; for worms and parasites, 35–36, 232, 244; wound salve, 245. See also herbs for the female reproductive system
herbalism, methods of, 1–2
herbs for the female reproductive system: for common ailments, 162–166; hormonal balance, 153; for menopause, 159–162; menses, 150–151, 164; strengthening glands, 148–149; support pregnancy, 154–158; tone and strengthen the uterus, 152

Herring's Law of Cure, 227
hiatal hernia, 41, 42
high blood pressure, 98
high blood sugar, 49–50
high cholesterol, 96–97
hormones: bone and joint deterioration and, 93; essential fatty acids and, 82; female, 147–148, 152–153; growth hormones in food, 17; imbalance of, 61, 140; list of primary endocrine glands, 145–146; male, 167–169; and mineral balance, 85
hydrocortisone, 137
hydrotherapy: during cleanse, 25, 65, 89; colon 31; hot and cold showers, 102, 205-206, 209; hot baths, 204; for the lungs, 109; salt scrubs and ice rubs, 210; sauna, 210; traditional use of, 207
hyperglycemia, 51
hypersensitive immunity, 139–141
hypertension, 98
hyperthyroidism, 172–173
hypoglycemia, 50
hypothermia, 245
hypothyroidism, 171–172

I

IBS (irritable bowel syndrome), 42, 44–45
ICF #1 / ICF #2 (American Botanical Pharmacy's Intestinal Formulas), 27–28, 34, 61
immune system: and asthma, 114; boosting the, 223–224; danger of growth hormones to the, 17; digestion linked to poor functioning, 49; echinacea as boost to, 242; emotions and the, 224; essential fatty acids and, 82; function of the, 213–214; herbal remedies for the, 24, 72, 218–221; innate or nonspecific immunity, 214; intestinal flora, 221–225; low acid levels in

stomach and poor, 42; managing illness, 226–229; specific of adaptive immunity, 215–217
incontinence, 134–135
indigestion, 43–44, 77–78, 245
infection, 107, 121–122
inflammation, 79, 82, 86–87, 93–94, 101, 113
injury treatment, 243–245
insect bites, 246
insomnia, 188–189, 245
insulin, 47, 51–52, 145
interferon, 215–216
internal bleeding, 243
interstitial cystitis, 135–136
intestinal flora, 236–237
intestinal system: appendix pain, 29–31; benefits of bowel cleansing, 13–14, 16–17, 24–29; colitis, 31–32; constipation, 32; diagram, 12; diarrhea, 33–34; diverticulitis, 34; function of the, 11, 13; intestinal flora, 221–224; large intestine, 14–16; the Revitalizing Diet, 17–21; small intestine, 14; worms and parasites, 34–37
iodine and thyroid balance, 171–173
iron, anemia and, 90–92
irritable bowel syndrome (IBS), 42, 44–45

J

jaundice, 70–71
joints, 49, 82, 93–94, 101

K

kidneys: and bone vitality, 85; care of the, 25, 126–127; foods that activate / cleanse, 127–128; function of the, 125–126; herbs that aid the, 98, 126–130, 244; influence on the circulatory system, 78, 98; and lymph care, 208; one-week cleanse, 130–133; skin and cleanse of the,

Index to Botanicals

The Author

Karin Christa Uphoff holds a bachelor of science degree from Oregon State University and a master's degree in zoology from Arizona State University. Having worked as a wildlife ecologist, animal behavior researcher, teacher, and environmental consultant, she undertook advanced training in massage therapy, vibrational medicine, and yoga, then earned a diploma in herbal medicine and natural healing in the UK. Her professional affiliations include the Pacific Environmental Education Center, the American Herbalist Association, the American Herbalist Guild, and United Plant Savers. Ms. Uphoff is a practicing herbalist, teacher, and nutritional consultant in northern California. Visit her website at www. rainbowconnection.net

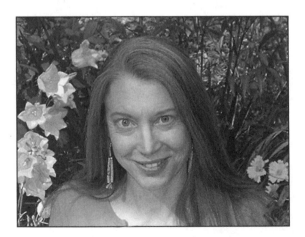